COLD LAND, WARM HEARTS

More Memories of an Arctic Medical Outpost

COLD LAND, WARM HEARTS

More Memories of an Arctic Medical Outpost

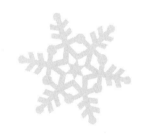

KEITH BILLINGTON

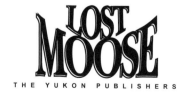

THE YUKON PUBLISHERS

Lost Moose is an imprint of Harbour Publishing Co. Ltd.
Harbour Publishing Co. Ltd.
P.O. Box 219, Madeira Park, BC, V0N 2H0
www.harbourpublishing.com

To protect the privacy of individuals, some names have been changed.
All photographs from the collection of Keith Billington unless noted otherwise.
Edited by Betty Keller
Maps by Roger Handling
Cover design by Teresa Karbashewski
Text design by Michelle Winegar
Printed and bound in Canada

 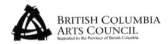

**Canada Council
for the Arts**

**Conseil des Arts
du Canada**

BRITISH COLUMBIA
ARTS COUNCIL
Supported by the Province of British Columbia

Harbour Publishing acknowledges financial support from the Government of
Canada through the Canada Book Fund and the Canada Council for the Arts,
and from the Province of British Columbia through the BC Arts Council and the
Book Publishing Tax Credit.

LIBRARY AND ARCHIVES CANADA CATALOGUING IN PUBLICATION
Billington, Keith, 1940-
     Cold land, warm hearts : more memories of an Arctic
medical outpost / Keith Billington.

ISBN 978-1-55017-534-9

     1. Billington, Keith, 1940-. 2. Billington, Muriel.
3. Nurses—Northwest Territories—Fort McPherson
Region—Biography. 4. Midwives—Northwest Territories—Fort
McPherson Region—Biography. 5. Gwich'in Indians—Social
life and customs. 6. Gwich'in Indians—Medical care—Northwest
Territories—Fort McPherson Region. 7. Medical care—Northwest
Territories—Fort McPherson Region—History—20th century.
8. Fort McPherson Region (N.W.T.) —Biography. I. Title.

RT37.B54A3 2010   610.73092   C2010-904449-5

To my children,
Helen, Stephen and David.

The end of a thing is better than the beginning—
Do not say, "Why were the former days better than these?"
For you do not inquire wisely concerning this.

Ecclesiastes 7:8–10

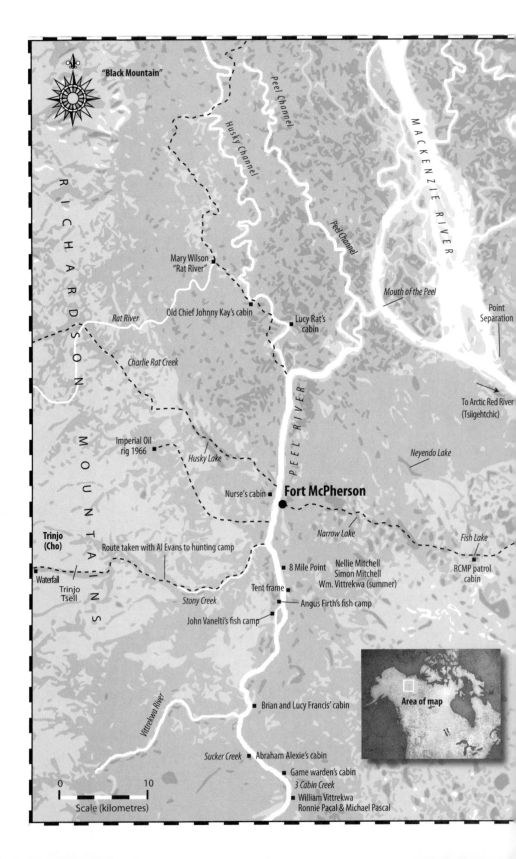

INTRODUCTION

THE GWICH'IN PEOPLE OF THE NORTHWEST TERRITORIES have been coping with change since white people first came to their land, and by and large they have adjusted remarkably well. But the decade ending in 1970 was the twilight of their traditional way of life as communication systems became more sophisticated and airports were constructed. Then in 1978 their isolation came to an abrupt end with the completion of the Dempster Highway, which snaked 740 kilometres across the tundra from Dawson City in the south, over the Ogilvie and Richardson mountains and through the Mackenzie Delta to arrive in Inuvik.

Adjusting to change was something that my wife, Muriel, and I had also done remarkably well when we went north in September 1963. Both registered nurses and in our early twenties, we had emigrated to Canada from England, and after an orientation year working at the Charles Camsell Indian and Eskimo Hospital in Edmonton, Alberta, we had flown north to the Gwich'in settlement of Fort McPherson, an isolated village on the southwestern edge of the Mackenzie Delta. We were responsible for the healthcare of all the residents there as well as those in Arctic Red River, a small village of one hundred people sixty-four kilometres to the east.

We sutured wounds, extracted teeth and prepared bodies for burial after tragic deaths. As Muriel was a nurse-midwife, she delivered many of the babies and taught me how to deliver them when

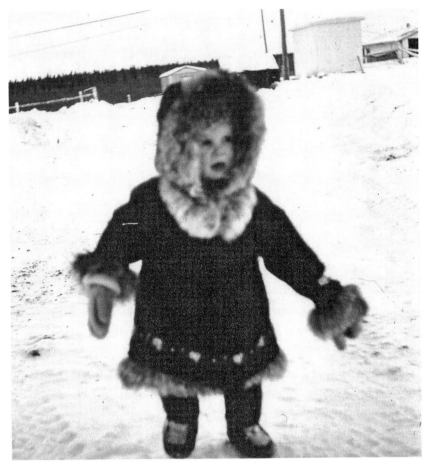

Stephen goes out for a stroll in his fur-trimmed parka.

she was away. And whenever emergencies were not occurring, we worked hard to develop a comprehensive public health program at the local school, in the village and in the hunting and trapping camps. Of course, we could not have functioned as well as we did without the capable help of a Gwich'in housekeeper—first Maria Itsi then Rachel Stuart and finally Mary Teya—and the nursing station's handyman—first William Firth and then Albert Peterson.

In the course of our six years at the nursing station we had two children, Helen and Stephen, who grew up accepting a life of cold winters, wearing mukluks and fur-trimmed parkas and travelling by

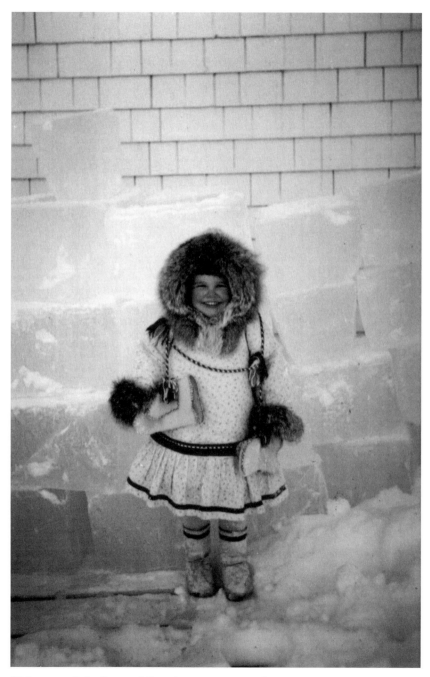

Helen stands in front of the winter water supply.

dog team. They relished the dry meat, dried fish and bannock that Mary Firth provided when she was babysitting them during the day. We developed close friendships with many of the Gwich'in people, but especially with William and Mary Firth, who became the children's surrogate grandfather (*jijii*) and grandmother (*jijuu*).

When it was finally time for us to move on, it was heart-rending to leave a place that had become home, so it wasn't surprising that fourteen years after leaving we made plans for a return visit. In the intervening time many old friends had died, and a visit to the graveyard was an emotional event for us. In 2009, twenty-six years after our first return visit, we made another trip to Fort McPherson, driving the well-maintained Dempster Highway. This time we were pleasantly surprised at some of the changes in the village but found that the Gwich'in people were still as friendly and hospitable as they had been so many years earlier. "Remember when …" became almost a mantra as we visited people who had grown older and perhaps wiser in the ways of the modern world. No one can visit a people or a place that has had a profound influence on his life without reminiscing about the old days, but as the pages of history were turned back, it was evident that "the good old days" of hardship and adventure had not always been so good, and changes had been inevitable and necessary for the Gwich'in.

Cold Land, Warm Hearts is the story of our return to a people, a place and a page of history.

CHAPTER ONE

CRACK! THE SOUND OF A RIFLE echoed around the Richardson Mountains. Muriel and I had been walking along a high shale bluff to watch some caribou, but now we stopped to listen. Crack! There it was again. The caribou looked up uneasily and then continued grazing, stepping over the grassy hillocks then stopping again to nibble some succulent piece of greenery.

"Someone must be shooting at the caribou." I stated the obvious.

Below us two small figures appeared around a grey shale outcrop, a common part of the landscape around Wrights Pass on the Dempster Highway. We watched as they slithered down the slope, each carrying a rifle slung over his back, then walked over the tundra with the peculiar gait that told us that their feet were sinking periodically into the water-filled holes that lie between the tufts of coarse grass and ground birch. They were headed for what we could now see was a young bull caribou lying on its side and almost hidden by a patch of ground birch. The animal must have been dawdling behind the rest of the small herd when the hunters spotted it, and a shot through the neck had brought it down.

Muriel and I hurried down from our viewpoint to our truck and drove along the road closer to where the kill had taken place. I could see that one of the hunters was a Gwich'in man whom I thought I recognized. Hastily putting on my boots, I walked over to where he was standing by the caribou. He had pulled out a knife with a saw attachment and began to saw the antlers off the animal. "Hi there, Abe!" I was guessing at his name because I wasn't sure. "Fancy meeting you up here. It's been a long time. How are you doing?"

"Hey! It's Keith, isn't it? What you doing up here?" We chatted for a while and he told me that his sister Rosie had passed away the previous year. Then he asked, "Are you going to the village? Come and see me later when I get back."

"What are you going to do with those?" I indicated the antlers that he was discarding.

"You can have them if you want. I only want the meat."

I thanked him and said I would visit with him later on. We chatted for a while then, having no desire to watch the animal being butchered, I took a photograph, picked up the antlers and headed back to the truck.

It was August 2009 and Muriel and I were on our way north from Dawson City, driving the 550 kilometres up the Dempster Highway—the "Last Adventure Highway in North America"—to revisit the village that had been our home for six years and the birthplace of two of our children. Fort McPherson, which today has a population of over eight hundred Gwich'in First Nations people, lies on the east bank of the Peel River, on the virtual edge of the Mackenzie Delta and within 20 kilometres of the barren, rolling foothills of the Richardson Mountains. It is 160 kilometres inside the Arctic Circle and 3,500 kilometres north of Vancouver, British Columbia. Since 1978 it has been joined by a narrow gravel road to Inuvik, 195 kilometres to the north.

Our anticipation and excitement at the prospect of seeing friends in Fort McPherson had been heightened by our experiences on the drive north. The Last Adventure Highway had lived up to its name. The scenery had been astounding as we passed the Tombstone Mountains and drove into the alpine tundra where a dozen different hues of red contrasted with the yellows and greens of the willow bushes and aspen trees. Towering over everything was the granite grey rock of the Ogilvie Mountains. One day we had observed a flock of perhaps 200,000 sandhill cranes travelling down the Tintina Trench to warmer climes. Another day it was a large "V" of geese flying south, while a few small lakes along the roadside provided temporary homes to ducks also on their way south. Although we had driven through some muddy sections, the highway hadn't been as bad as we'd been led to expect, and as we climbed higher the road conditions improved. Here the spectacular colours of bearberry, dwarf birch and willow contrasted with the duller red of fireweed as it went rapidly to seed. I stopped our truck suddenly when we spotted two caribou standing majestically on the brow of a hill, their large antlers held high as they watched us, and then a few minutes later we were amazed to see a small herd of caribou being followed by not one but five grizzly bears! One grizzly had finished hunting for the day and was lying belly down on top of the caribou kill on which he had gorged himself. We knew he was a large silvertip, although all we could see of him as he lay sprawled out on his bloody kill was his back, which shone alternately light and dark as the sunlight played to his rhythmic breathing.

Not too far away another drama was being acted out. A sow grizzly with two cubs was being stalked by a large male—males are known to kill and eat cubs—and as we watched, the sow stopped periodically and chased the big male for a short distance then returned to her cubs and continued walking up the hillside. Soon the male would start following again, getting ever closer until at last the sow had obviously had enough of this game. She suddenly swung around and with surprising speed ran down the hill straight at the annoying male. He came to a sudden stop and then turned and ran off down the hill without any dignity at all. Only when he was far enough away did the sow return to her young.

The fifth grizzly was a sly one, walking along in the same direction as the caribou as though dinner was the last thing on his mind. He was in no hurry, stopping to nibble on some morsel on the ground from time to time before setting off again, but always in the

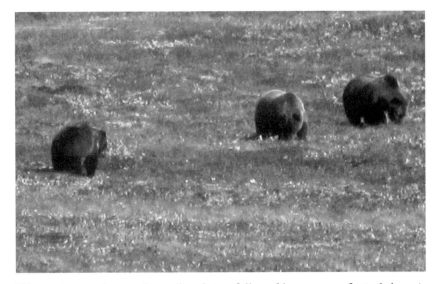

We were amazed to see the caribou being followed by a group of grizzly bears!

same direction as the caribou. They were very aware of the grizzly, pausing to look over toward him, then grazing for a second or two before walking relentlessly on. And at last we were reminded that we too had to keep going if we wanted to reach our destination.

As we drove along the gravel highway, we saw more small herds of caribou continuing their northward trek to the calving grounds, moving steadily over the tundra, keeping to the low ground where there was a lot of feed and very few annoying flies. I found myself looking out over that bleak and vast panorama and wondering which of the surrounding mountains I had travelled over with my dog team when I had visited the Gwich'in hunting camps. And then suddenly my mind was filled with pictures of the time that I had gone with a group of Gwich'in men on a caribou hunt.

The ubiquitous moccasin telegraph had brought the welcome news that the annual migration of caribou had begun in the Richardson Mountains, and as caribou was the Gwich'in's main source of protein, they had immediately begun preparing their dog teams to go hunting. It would take several days by sled to reach the vicinity of the caribou, camping and hunting would take many weeks and then

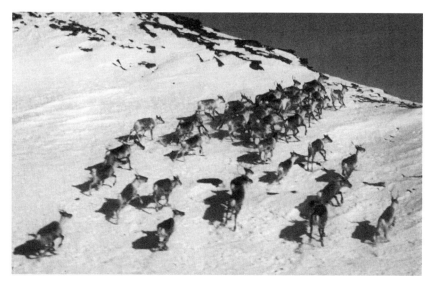

A small group of caribou run to join the 65,000 strong Porcupine herd in the Richardson Mountains. FRANK DUNN PHOTO.

hauling the meat home would take another few days. Soon several Gwich'in families set off for the Richardson Mountains and others came to our clinic for first aid supplies as they prepared to follow them to the caribou meat camps.

In those days I had not needed too much of an invitation to travel to the camps, and when several people told me that it would be good idea to go and make sure everyone was okay, I conferred with my long-suffering wife. Muriel said that she didn't mind staying home with our children, Helen and Stephen, who were now four and two years old respectively, and we knew that our neighbour and friend Mary Firth would look after them during the day when Muriel was working in the nursing station. "After all," she said, "we know that one or two of the women are pregnant, and there may be others we don't know about. Besides, most of the families will be up in the camps, so why not go?" Then she added, "But I'd feel better if someone went with you."

I visited the RCMP barracks to tell the Mounties of my plans and asked Constable Al Evans if he knew of anyone who was available to go. "I don't particularly want to go on several days' journey into the mountains on my own," I explained.

His eyes brightened as he told me that by pure coincidence his corporal had suggested that he visit some of the camps for liaison purposes and for general interest as well—if he could find someone to go with him. "So would it be okay if we went together? That way everyone will be satisfied." It wasn't long before we were spreading maps over his office desk and poring over the section where I had been told we could expect to find the hunters. We made plans to leave at the weekend and return after a few days at the camps.

I gathered the food supplies I would need, and that evening Muriel cooked a large pile of donuts for me to take. But when she tasted one, she said that the fat had not been hot enough and they had absorbed too much of it. "Never mind," I said, relishing the one that I was eating. "I won't know the difference when I'm in the mountains!"

Trying to anticipate what I might need to take for the families in camp, I packed boxes of medical and dental supplies in my sleeping bag then added extra clothes, food and dog feed, an axe, matches, a canvas tent and a wood stove and stowed it all on my toboggan. When everything was ready and the dogs hitched up, I put the dog chains into a bag and stashed them where I could easily locate them at the end of the day on the trail. I kissed Muriel good-bye, stepped on the back of the toboggan, and at my cry of "Let's go!" the dogs hurtled out of the nursing station yard toward the river where Al Evans joined me with his team. We travelled south for four and a half kilometres to the mouth of Stoney Creek where we turned and started following it up to its source.

Stoney Creek is well named, and every toboggan that had been hauled up it had left some slivers of wood on the sharp rocks that jutted up through the ice. The scenery changed with every bend, and though it was like many other creeks I had travelled on, it seemed particularly beautiful as the sun shone down on the bluffs rising on either side of us. In one section thirty-metre high banks were covered with a profusion of spruce and birch trees. Around another bend the trees disappeared, the cliffs shot up to 125 metres, and the sharp particles of shale they spit out into the wind landed on the ice where they caught under the toboggans, making it difficult for the dogs to pull them. We passed piles of huge sandstone blocks, which must have weighed several hundred kilograms and looked as though some giant hand had placed them one on top of the other. High above them and silhouetted against a deep blue sky, half a dozen ravens played in the wind currents. Later in the day as we travelled toward the setting sun, we could hear gusts of wind blowing across the top of the creek banks high above us and little flurries of snow would drift down through the still air and settle in the creek bed.

By dusk Al and I had arrived at a traditional stopping place called Trinjo on the edge of the foothills where there were good spruce boughs to be found for our tent floor and dry wood for the stove. As we worked to put up the tent and cut enough firewood to last the night, a full moon began to rise above us, so by the time our chores were done and the dogs fed, it seemed as bright as day. The dogs sighed with comfort as they settled their full stomachs down on a bed of spruce branches, and everywhere became absolutely still and quiet.

Early the next morning, feeling quite refreshed after a good night's sleep, we broke camp and continued up the creek. It was now covered with a couple of centimetres of snow, which had fallen after the creek had overflowed and refrozen, and the dogs had no difficulty pulling our loaded toboggans. At intervals we passed huge, turquoise-coloured bumps on the creek ice, which we thought must be about to explode or collapse because the ice sounded very hollow as the sleds sped by, but nothing happened and the humps were still there when we came past on our way home several days later.

At the headwaters of Stoney Creek we came to an inhospitable place that the Gwich'in called Brass House. It was devoid of trees and the only life apparent in the icy panorama were some young willows that were locked in the frozen embrace of newly formed ice. Here the wind was relentless and seemed to be making up for the time it had been unable to reach us when we were protected by the recesses of the creek. It now seemed to be blowing right through our winter clothes. Later it was explained to me that a man called Brass had lived in a small cabin here, probably during the push to reach the Yukon goldfields, but as with many dozens of other gold seekers, no one knew what had become of him.

We climbed toward higher ground where the snow was much deeper and hard packed by the wind, and when we looked up at the mountains, we saw that they too were covered in ice and snow. There were now many small frozen channels funnelling into the main creek and draining the surrounding tundra. As we stopped to rest the dogs and look around through our frost-encrusted parkas, we saw that in several places the water had forced its way over the surface of the ice and was freezing in great brownish grey expanses, which still steamed where they came in contact with the frigid air. We saw a tent that was pitched beside the creek where water from a collapsed ice bulge had suddenly flooded one area. Some unfortunate and weary traveller had obviously decided to wait here for the ice to become firm enough to travel on, and because of the lack of trees at this point, he had used armfuls of thin willows for the tent floor. We would have paused here to make a meal, but as the stove looked as though it was on the verge of collapse, we only stopped for a few minutes before pushing on.

We began climbing steadily toward a distant mountain pass, and as we climbed the temperature dropped in spite of the brilliant sunshine. However, the dogs pulled well, their effort apparent by the steam that rose from them and the resulting frost that adhered to their coats. Al and I kept warm by pushing the toboggans up the hill in order to help the dogs, but the scarves covering our noses and chins became heavily encrusted with ice. Passing over a small knoll, we descended into a shallow hidden valley, aptly called "The Shute." It was perhaps a kilometre long, and at its far end we could see that the dog team trail we were following continued up the mountain. As we rode along, we saw pieces of caribou bones and scraps of hide beside a small, burnt-out campfire where Gwich'in hunters had no doubt stopped for tea or a meal, but we pressed on in the hope that we would soon get some relief from the wind.

Whenever I am driving dogs, or for that matter whenever I am out walking in a park, I glance behind me periodically. I suppose I expect to be attacked by wolves or a bear, but even knowing that this is foolish, I always feel better if I glance back. So while I was travelling behind Al, during one of these quick glances I noticed that there was something following us. I hailed Al and we both stopped. It was a dog, a sled dog, but where he had come from we didn't have a clue. He wouldn't approach us when we stopped and called to him, but after that this skinny loner continued to follow us slowly up the hills and along the creeks. When we finally lost sight of him, we figured that he had been just too tired to make the last couple of kilometres, and I knew how he must have felt as I looked ahead and saw that the trail kept going up and up as far as the eye could see.

At first the climb wasn't too bad, although the dogs were already straining to pull the load so there was no way we could even think of riding. However, I soon found that there is a limit to how long one can jog uphill behind a toboggan. After a few kilometres of this, the trail went up the mountainside so steeply that we had to help push the toboggans. By this time we had climbed nearly a thousand metres, and our breath was coming in short gasps as we pushed and shouted encouragement to the dogs. We stopped every few hundred metres, sat on our loads and crammed some of Muriel's incredibly fatty, sweet, frozen doughnuts into our mouths. As this seemed to be exactly what our bodies needed, I was so glad they had been failures!

The nearer we got to the summit, the less snow there was because it had been blown from the rocks by the high winds. In fact, the winds are so strong in this area that back in the 1940s a man and his dog team had been blown off one of these mountains and not found until the following spring. With no shelter to hide in or tree to hang onto when the winds are blowing at over three hundred kilometres an hour, it was easy to see how this could happen. Fortunately for Al and me, the winds we had experienced lower down had now died, and the air was so calm that we could see clearly through the frigid air.

When we stopped for a short rest at the top of the pass, we soon felt the cold seeping into our sweaty clothes and starting to freeze them, so we were forced to go on. We shouted to the dogs, and they got up, shook themselves and seemed eager to go, so perhaps they were also feeling the cold. The wind had deposited deep snow on the downhill track, and the dogs now ran along with their tails held high as though they were really enjoying themselves because gravity was doing the work for them, but I had to ride my brake most of the way so that the toboggan wouldn't rear-end my wheel dog. This brake consisted of a curved piece of metal welded to a large hinge; when not in use, the brake was kicked up onto the riding platform. When needed, it was kicked down and the driver stood on it with varying degrees of pressure to slow down the sled.

It did not take long to reach the bottom and we stopped in the shelter of some scrubby trees to catch our breath but decided against lighting a fire. Although we hadn't seen any caribou or sled tracks, we felt that we must be very close to a hunting camp. A few minutes later we suddenly emerged from a tight stand of spruce trees onto a trail that had been hacked through willow bushes two and three metres high. These willows were quite dangerous because, as the toboggan went over them, they sprang back, hitting us on the unprotected portions of our anatomy. The ground birch that we went through was equally annoying for the dogs as it pulled at their faces, but they kept persistently on, perhaps smelling caribou ahead.

By now it was getting dark. As the bright moon started to show its face, the snow-covered mountains around us looked very bleak, and though I had a travelling companion with me, it felt very lonely out there. Then to our consternation, as we came out of the willow grove we saw that the trail took another upward swing over a small pass. We could do nothing but follow it. I felt myself withdrawing into my parka and I began working like an automaton, jogging sometimes and riding whenever the trail was level. I tried not to look too far ahead because it was usually disappointing to see the trail still stretching out ahead of us in the moonlight.

From the top of the pass, the trail wound down toward another creek. Al gave me a few minutes head start so that his team would not run into mine, and I was glad that he did because the trail got steeper and steeper. I made all sorts of chirps and whistles to keep my team going, since I could hardly see my lead dog in the shadows of the narrow creek. Glancing back, I saw that Al's team was already snaking down the trail toward me, and I shouted for my dogs to get a move on.

Suddenly there was a hefty bump and I nearly let go of the handlebars as they twisted in my grip. The toboggan had dropped about one and a half metres onto another frozen streambed, skirted around an old stump or boulder—I wasn't sure which—and then as the dogs' harness tightened and they strained ahead, the toboggan popped up the side of the obstruction and ran smoothly onto the trail again.

There were now several trails leading off from the main one, but since my leader carried on as if he knew exactly where he was going, I let him take the initiative. He soon stopped by an empty tent and immediately started to tear at an old piece of caribou hide that was lying there. I knew the dogs had worked very hard and were ravenously hungry, but in case a fight developed I kicked the piece of hide away into the distance. As I did so, I thought that I could hear some dogs barking in the distance. Great! We were nearly at an inhabited camp with real live people! I turned to look for Al and saw his dogs rounding the bend in the trail, the team spaced out neatly. "There are some dogs over there, Al. Maybe we can camp with the owners," I called.

No answer.

"Al!" I yelled, then added quickly as Al's dogs reached me, "Whoa, you idiots!"

Al's five dogs stopped and lay down, but to my utter amazement and astonishment there was no sign of Al or his toboggan! I looked at the ends of the harness where the toboggan should have been and saw that the leather was torn.

"You stupid dogs, where on earth is Al?" I knew it was pointless to ask them, but talking to them stopped me from talking to myself.

I told my dogs to sit, though they didn't need telling. Then with muttered curses I turned Al's reluctant dogs around, took hold of the broken ends of the harness in my hands as if I was driving a horse, and trotted up the trail behind the dogs. If some of my Gwich'in friends had seen me, they would have been convulsed with laughter. On the other hand, one of the old men—someone like Peter Thompson—would not have looked surprised at all but simply raised his hat and said, "Good evening, Mr. Billington." But here I was, far away from any seeing eyes, still feeling self-conscious as I ran along the trail with an invisible toboggan.

Then through the gloom I saw the outline of Al, his back bent double, pushing his toboggan along the trail. What a pair we must have looked, Al with a dogless toboggan and me with a toboggan-less dog team. I must have been very tired and a little light-headed from all the work and little food because the whole thing suddenly struck me as very funny and I began to laugh and laugh. Al couldn't help laughing too, and it was not until we had sufficiently recovered that he told me what had happened. Like me, he had dropped into the little cross-creek and his dogs had shot out and around the rock, but his toboggan had hooked on it and the stitching gave way on the harness.

In the darkness we fixed up the harnesses as best as we could, then with me riding on top of the load and Al on behind, we came back to where my dogs were waiting. My youngest dog, Thursday, had somehow managed to get out of his harness, but he hadn't fought with any of the other dogs and came as soon as I called him. Minutes later we were on our way again toward the sounds of barking dogs, and in what seemed like no time at all we saw the glow of a candle-lit tent ahead.

"Who's there?" a voice called out and I recognized it as belonging to William Smith, a tall Gwich'in man from Fort McPherson.

"It's Keith. And Al Evans," I called back, and then turning to Al I said, "We'll tie the dogs up over by those trees so they won't bother anyone's stuff."

"Come on in when you've tied your dogs. You must be tired after that trip!" Then William laughed, and I wondered if he was pulling our legs, because most white people did not travel that far out into the bush.

William and his wife, Charlotte, had a big canvas tent and intended to stay where they were for a few weeks. He had shot some caribou and a moose and they had been busy cutting up the meat and drying it. A wooden frame within the tent held strips of thinly cut moose and caribou meat, and the smell of drying meat mixed with that of woodsmoke and spruce boughs. Charlotte had made a quantity of "itsoo," desiccated dry meat mixed with flour, sugar and berries and then rolled into balls with melted fat.

They invited us to stay with them for the night, and we appreciated the invitation for it meant not having to put up our tent after our hard day on the trail or even to utilize the empty tent that we had passed a little way back. Charlotte fried some meat for us and served it with large pieces of bannock. William traded us some meat for some of the commercial dog mush that we had brought, and this enabled us to feed our dogs quickly with a more satisfying meal. As it was now quite late, it didn't take us long to climb into our sleeping bags and fall fast asleep.

The noise of clattering pots and pans woke me in the morning. Charlotte was already cooking breakfast. William, who was the first up, had lit the fire in the stove and was coming into the tent with an armful of firewood. Al was just sitting up and rubbing his eyes so I didn't feel that I was the only lazy lodger. Charlotte cooked pancakes, which she served with butter and sugar and a good hunk of fried caribou meat, and we all sat around the stove on our rolled-up sleeping bags munching away and sipping scalding hot tea. Afterwards Al mended his harness traces using copper rivets and a roll of babiche to fasten the leather securely to the rings and clips.

"How are your hands?" I asked Charlotte. She had some deformed fingers, which may have been frostbitten when she was young, and now she suffered with some arthritis in the joints during the cold weather.

"Oh, they're okay, I guess. I have to cut up this meat anyway so I just take a pain pill if they get too bad." She indicated the moose hindquarters lying on some spruce brush in the corner of the tent. "When the meat is cold, it's hard for me to do but I like it after!" She nodded toward the meat drying on the racks.

William was going to go up the mountain to pick up some caribou he had shot the previous day and invited us along. "There might be part of another herd close by you can see," he told us.

Charlotte had told me earlier that there were a few people a short way off who would probably like to see me and get some medicine, but I wanted to take William up on his offer. "Charlotte," I said, "if you see any of the other people, will you tell them I'll see them later in the day if they want?"

Al and I packed rifles, snowshoes, lunch and tea but left our other things in the tent so our dogs would have no difficulty pulling us up the first hill and over the gradually rising tundra. I also left my dog Thursday at the camp because he yapped a lot and might scare the caribou away. On the windward side of the mountain the going was quite rough and bumpy because the snow had been blown off the tussocks of coarse grass and moss. On the lee side there was much more snow, and as it had been packed down by the wind, the route was smooth and easy. We saw the hoof marks and trails of what must have been thousands of caribou that had passed that way. We could see where they had scratched away the snow to reveal the lichens on which they browsed, and bloodstains on the snow indicated where a caribou had been shot. In some places the antlers were still lying there because the Gwich'in priority was for the edible parts that could be eaten by both man or beast.

William Smith was leading the way and he pointed to a small rise about four hundred metres to his right where a black wolf was running up the hillside. It stopped for a moment, looked at us over its shoulder and then took off again, disappearing over the brow of the hill. We drove our teams over to the hill and, examining the huge footprint the wolf had left in a patch of soft snow, realized that it must have weighed at least fifty-four kilograms. But William was annoyed when we came to where his caribou were and saw that the wolf had eaten a large portion of two of them. However, as the carcasses were still good for dog feed, he started to load them to take back to camp before the wolf came back to finish his meal. Meanwhile, as more caribou tracks led toward the other side of the mountain, Al and I decided that we would go on a little bit further.

When we came to a place where a few scrub willows grew, we tied up the dogs and, shouldering our rifles and snowshoes, continued walking over the wind-packed snow. The sun was high now but the wind was very cold, and as we walked from each sheltered area into an exposed area, we alternated between being very hot and sweaty to feeling half-frozen, though both were bearable as long as we kept walking. There were no signs of live caribou, but here and there were flattened, bloodstained patches in the snow showing that the hunters had been there a few days earlier, and as we scanned the area we could see antlers sticking up out of the snow as a reminder that another animal had met man.

The sky was an incredible blue with a few clouds scudding across the Mackenzie Delta, and Al and I climbed to a hilltop and sat down with our backs to the wind to survey the landscape that stretched below us. From here we could see how the myriad caribou tracks had formed some sort of order about a kilometre away before they funneled off northward. While we ate the bannock and meat that Charlotte had given us, we noticed that Gwich'in hunters had shot six caribou nearby then laid them side by side, propped up on their eviscerated bellies so they would drain and the meat would cool. Around the carcasses sticks had been poked into the snow and string fastened to them from which bits of cloth, cigarette packages and spent 30-30 and .303 cartridges had been suspended. These were to keep away the ravens and the wolves, who preferred the same delicacies as the Gwich'in—the eyes, brain, heart, liver and kidneys.

We decided that we should start back or we would be as cold as the caribou carcasses, and we were thirsty and had left the tea in our dogsleds. We came back down the mountain to where the dogs were and, after gathering a few handfuls of dead willows, made a fire to melt some snow in the metal billycan to make some strong sweet tea. Then as it was getting colder by the minute, we untangled the dogs and headed for camp. Our dogs had no difficulty following the fresh scent of William's dogs and an hour and a half later we were sitting in William and Charlotte's tent sharing more tea and the meal of fried moose meat that Charlotte had cooked for us. While we were eating, William fed our dogs, so between him and his wife we felt that we were being treated regally. They told us that since the caribou had moved further north, some of the people who had been camping a few kilometres away had moved on, leaving the caribou we had seen on the mountain for William, and this would give him all the meat he would need.

I put on my snowshoes, picked up my medical bag and walked down the trail for about a kilometre, turning there toward a canvas tent where the stove was belching out a lot of smoke. I knocked on the tent frame to announce my presence and a voice shouted out, "Come in!" I pulled aside the heavy piece of material that acted as a door and went in, ducking my head slightly as I entered and straightening up once inside. I was always surprised how high these tents were set. There were several people gathered inside, and as soon as I sat down on a rolled eiderdown, I was handed a cup of tea.

I was told, "There's only us here now. The others have gone further up to get more caribou. We will go up tomorrow or tomorrow next day," which was the Gwich'in way of saying "the day after tomorrow," but I thought it was equally descriptive.

After talking with them about how they were doing, one old lady asked if I had any pain pills with me, as she had left hers at home. "I'll leave you a few for now," I told her, "but ask one of the young guys who are going to town with meat to bring your pills up for you."

"Aha!" she said as she took the small container of pills from me."

After seeing all the knives around and noticing small cuts on some of the women's hands, I asked if they had brought Band-Aids with them.

"Not many."

"Well, here's a package, but try to clean your hands of all that blood before you put one on. You don't want to get an infection while you're up here."

Everyone was quite healthy, and it came to me as I walked back to William and Charlotte's tent—as it had on earlier visits to the camps—that when the people were out on the land, they seemed much happier than when they were in town.

That night Al and I decided that instead of going on, we should start for home the following morning because we would have two hard days' travel ahead of us. We turned in early and lay in our bags listening to Radio Station CHAK from Inuvik and watching the red glow from the stove reflecting on the tent walls. It was a great feeling but one that could not be enjoyed for long because its hypnotic effect soon had us nodding off to sleep.

At first light we started packing even as William was lighting the stove and Charlotte was getting breakfast ready. As we turned the toboggans upright and started to carry our belongings out of the tent, the dogs perked up, and by the time we began stretching out their harnesses, they were jumping up and down and barking in anticipation. We said thank you and goodbye to our hosts and set off on the trail for home. It had been a good visit, and I felt that I had come to know William and Charlotte a bit better. When they were in the village, they lived in a tiny house with their two teenage children. We saw the children at the school and in the hostel for routine health exams, but we rarely saw their parents.

As we retraced our steps homeward, we were soon lathered in sweat. The hills that had been such a relief to us as we headed for the camp now turned their backs on us, and we had to struggle up them, shouting encouragement to the dogs whenever we had enough breath to do so. But we laughed as we passed the place where Al's toboggan and his dogs had parted company.

Climbing toward the high pass that would lead us to the Shute and then the headwaters of Stoney Creek, Al spotted a flock of ptarmigan, their pure white colouring making them almost invisible against the snow. What had caught his eye was that they kept flying up and then coming back down just a few metres further on. But it wasn't our presence that was making them nervous—a wolf was stalking the birds. We stopped our dogs to watch. The wolf, a large grey and white animal, lay on his stomach watching the birds then creeping slowly forward on his belly. Each time they spotted him, the birds would take flight then land close by again. When we started walking slowly ahead to keep this fascinating behaviour in view, we spotted another wolf, smaller but with the same colouring, lying behind a bush toward which the ptarmigan were being herded.

When at last the first wolf realized that he was being watched by us, he ran across a small creek where he was joined by the other wolf and they both raced for the face of one of the mountains. Without pausing they ran rapidly up the incredibly steep mountainside and only slowed when they were mere specks against the snowy back-drop. I watched them through the scope on my rifle until they loped out of sight knowing that they were safe. I couldn't get over what a wonderful sight they were and how fortunate we had been to see the smart moves they used to catch birds. We stayed a little longer to watch the ptarmigan, then as we couldn't hunt them because we only had high-powered rifles that would reduce a bird to feathers and splintered bone, we put our rifles away and continued the long arduous climb to the top of the pass.

We had been warned by the Gwich'in not to attempt to cross this pass if it was at all windy, and we were happy to see that it was not windy now, but while we had been visiting the camps, the wind had blown all the trail marks away. In fact, the snow was so clean and hard that I began to suspect that we were on the wrong pass. Then just as I had almost convinced myself that this was the case, I caught sight of an empty, very red ten-gallon gas drum, which up at this location and elevation looked incongruous. However, I had seen it on our way up, and Al had suggested that it may have been left by some geologist who did not want to carry it back or by a helicopter pilot doing survey work. Certainly no snowmobile had been up the mountain because back then they were not trusted too far from the village and especially up in the mountains.

We rested momentarily when we reached the top and enjoyed the fantastic view of mountains and valleys, all untouched by mankind. There was no pollution and, except for the two of us and the gas drum, no signs of civilization. My camera had frozen solid and I used Al's to take a picture of him before I began to feel the same as my camera as my sweat began to freeze in the frigid air.

Going down the other side of the pass was quite a feat because the toboggan brakes could not get a purchase on the rocks and ice, and we were in continual danger of running over the dogs. I could feel the rocks gouging out the bottom of the toboggan but there was no way we could stop, and as a result, we reached the bottom in a little more than half an hour, considerably faster than when we went up. It was much warmer in the creek valley, and as we meandered along, we relaxed and enjoyed ourselves again. Around three in the afternoon we stopped at an old campfire, made a fire and ate our lunch. Again we saw the stray dog but we could not entice him to come close, and even the food scraps that we put out some distance from us did not tempt him. We knew we should have shot him, but neither of us had the heart to kill this lonely animal. (Some days after our arrival home we learned that returning hunters had shot the dog to save it from being attacked and eaten by wolves. They were surprised that the wolves hadn't already got him, but that was possibly because caribou were so easily available to them.)

A few kilometres further down the creek we saw that the trail climbed again. I had been told that it detoured here to skirt a frozen waterfall, and I was curious to see what it looked like. I had also been told that someone had come up it with an empty toboggan, and I figured that if someone could get up it, we could get down it. We turned off the trail to follow the creek bed, going slowly in case we came suddenly to the waterfall. When I finally caught sight of it ahead, I stopped the dogs, which was when I discovered that the toboggan brake was not very effective on the ice, and as there was hardly any snow on the icy creek leading to the falls, our toboggans were quite eager to slide down the creek on their own without any help from the dogs. I solved the problem by tying my toboggan to Al's lead dog, and thankfully my dogs seemed content to lie down while I went ahead to check out the falls.

Concerned that my mukluks might slip on the ice, I climbed carefully down the one-metre drop to the head of the falls, making good use of the handhold provided by a few straggly willows. There was a rocky outcrop at the top, but I decided that if the toboggans were heeled over a bit as we went down, there should be no problem. The land flattened out a bit below the falls and I knew that there would be whitewater there in the summertime, but I didn't think it would be a problem for us as there was sufficient snow alongside the creek to slow the toboggans. I climbed up the icefall again and asked Al to keep a good strong hold on his dogs in case they took off after mine, knowing that if my toboggan got stuck and his team came down on top of mine, we would be in an awful mess.

I managed to get my dogs to the top of the icefall, then, tipping the toboggan on its side and trying to control the dogs from pulling too vigorously, I edged forward. Unfortunately, the ice was too slippery for me to hold the toboggan back, and it gained speed, hit a rock—which righted it—and then the handlebars struck the rock overhang. Normally it would have been jammed into that position but now the dogs were pulling forward down the icefall. There was the sound of splitting wood. Crack! And the toboggan shot down the ice. Oh no! I thought. It's going to be wrecked! "WHOA! WHOA!" I yelled, and surprisingly the dogs slithered to a stop at the bottom of the icefall. A moment later the toboggan crashed into my poor wheel dog.

I slid down the icefall and examined what I thought was bound to be a wrecked sleigh. The handlebar on one side had split as had a board on the bottom, but the damage was far less than I expected, and with care I would be able to get home without having to make major repairs. I went back to the icefall, and we managed to get Al's team down without incident.

Our goal that day was to reach Trinjo before making camp because there was firewood there and brush would be available for the tent floor, but it was still a long way off. Fortunately, just past the waterfall and canyon the other trail—the one that we should have taken—came down to meet Stoney Creek again, and there was the small tent set amid the willows that we had passed on the way up. Thinking that it fitted the saying "any port in a storm" and knowing there was a stove inside, we stopped to light a fire to try to get warm and make some tea. But the tent was so poorly set that we could barely sit up in it and the stove smoked so badly we had to vacate it until the air cleared. Then as we were settling down again, the heat from the stove melted the snow under it, causing the stove to sink down enough to bring the stove pipe into contact with the tent, and the canvas started to smoulder, making even more smoke. We quickly extinguished the fire with a handful of snow, but the willows on the floor of the tent were so uncomfortable that we voted it as the worst tea break that we had ever had, even though it had been a relief to crawl into that smoky environment to shelter from the biting wind. If the tent had been at all comfortable and if wood had been available for a prolonged fire, we would have contemplated staying there as we were tired and it was now getting dark.

However, we half reluctantly started down Stoney Creek again. We were soon travelling in the darkness but the dogs were able to follow the trail without difficulty, and we rode the toboggans huddled into our parkas against the cold wind, the silence and the dark. My lead dog, Silver, didn't need much encouragement at night, trotting on without me speaking to him, and I noticed that none of the dogs even stopped to relieve themselves during night travel, perhaps realizing that the faster they moved the sooner they would be able to eat and rest, which is what I was feeling as well by that time. Then suddenly, just as we were entering a canyon, Silver veered off the trail onto a gravel bar. Sometimes, I thought, that dog is very stupid. I could only make out the white blur of his tail, though he was a mere five or six metres in front of me, because the moon, which was just rising, cast a deep shadow ahead. I had just realized that the toboggan was being pulled over some jagged rocks when one of them caught on the second dog's harness and all the dogs stopped. I jumped off to find out what was wrong and immediately felt water seep into my mukluks. I leapt for the rocks, yelling "Overflow!" so that Al could stop his dogs before he got into it, too. Silver wasn't so stupid after all!

Although I knew that overflow on many of the northern creeks can make travel at night by dogsled very difficult, neither Al nor I had given it a thought. I knew that Vittrekwa Creek, thirty-two kilometres south of Stoney Creek, was the most notorious for ice and overflow, but I didn't know that the overflow on Stoney Creek occurs in the canyons when the water, under the ice and under pressure, suddenly bursts to the surface. It can flood the canyon from wall to wall, sometimes to a depth of many metres though at other times it may be only fifteen or twenty centimetres deep. I had heard the story of one of the young Gwich'in men who had been travelling alone when he was caught in a sudden overflow and he and his dogs had to swim for their lives.

Now, splashing through ankle-deep water, I led Silver to the end of the rocks and went back to discuss the situation with Al. There was no way we could stay where we were, and even though we had brought a tent, there was no place to set it and no brush available for flooring or wood for a fire. Although we couldn't see anything, we could hear the ice on our side crackling as the water covered it, so we decided that we would try to cross to the other side of the creek to see if it was free of water. But we knew that once we left the safety of the rocks we would have to go on because it would be impossible to turn the dogs around in the canyon. Balancing on a large rock, I quickly changed into dry footwear before my feet froze. I put my moccasin rubbers on then I went carefully to where Silver was standing and examined his feet. He seemed to be okay, but he was reluctant to start out because he had to step into the water, and more than ever before I knew I had to impress my will onto his mind. Taking out my whip, I cracked it ominously. "ALRIGHT!" I yelled. "GEE!" Silver obediently turned to the left and headed across the creek. I suspended myself on the lazyback so that my feet were not in the water, hoping that it would bear my weight after cracking at the icefall. Al stayed close behind so that his leader, who was a bit shy of the water, would follow me closely.

Once we got to the other side of the creek, I let Silver find his own way through the water. I kept encouraging him with shouts and a periodic crack of the whip, although I don't think that he needed any encouragement to find the driest route. I could hear the water rushing underneath the toboggan and at one point, as I felt it begin to float, I was filled with dread, but moments later Silver pulled to the right and I felt rather than saw that we were now gliding across ice again. After this little incident everything seemed to brighten up. We came out of the canyon, the moon shone brightly, the wind dropped, and we stopped to clean the ice from each of the dogs' feet and from the bottom of the toboggan. At about ten o'clock we arrived at Trinjo where we set the tent up by moonlight. There was firewood available so all we had to do was cut and split it. We fed the dogs and made some supper. As we crawled exhausted into our sleeping bags, we noted that it was one-thirty in the morning.

We didn't wake until nine but it didn't take us long to eat breakfast, pack, hitch up the dogs and get moving. The day was sunny and calm and the creek seemed to catch every ray of the sun. The

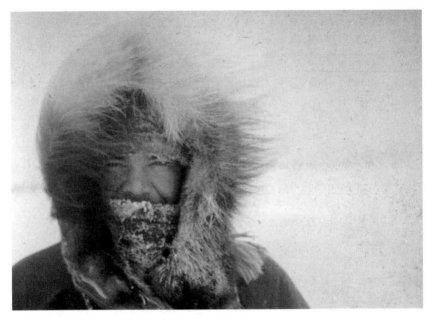

I look cold and windswept while travelling up the Peel River. M. WIGGINS
PHOTO.

dogs worked well and the toboggans moved easily, and as we went
through the portages close to the Peel River, I was careful not to pull
on the cracked handlebars, which had been getting steadily looser,
probably from my hanging on to them when I was going through
the water the previous night.

We arrived back in the village in the early afternoon, and as I enjoyed the comforts of home and told Muriel my story, the difficulties
of the trip faded away. It was Muriel who gently reminded me that
what was an adventure for me was everyday life for the Gwich'in.

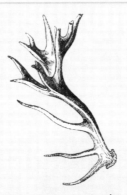

WHEN WHITE MEN CAME TO THIS area in the early 1800s, the Tetlit Gwich'in, or "Peel River People," had been living mostly in the wilderness of mountains, tundra and rivers that is now called the Yukon. When the deep snows melted in April and May, these people would migrate down to the rivers to set homemade nets in the eddies where there was an abundance of fish—whitefish, inconnu, crooked backs, grayling and arctic char. They dried these for use later in the year, making caches of them and of dried caribou meat up and down the country for use in hard times. Having an excellent knowledge of the country, they always knew where their own caches were, and they also knew that they would be left undisturbed by other people passing by.

When the Gwich'in travelled downriver, they packed their families, dogs and household goods into large moosehide-covered boats, using as many as sixteen untanned skins to make one boat, and using large sweeps to guide their boats as they floated down with the current. They were reluctant to travel all the way down the Peel River to its mouth because that area was a sort of no man's land between the Gwich'in and the Eskimo. When these two peoples did meet, they would fight, and it was often a take-no-prisoners war where men, women and children were slaughtered, although sometimes prisoners were taken as slaves.

When John Bell, who was in charge of the Hudson's Bay Company post in Fort Good Hope, came to trade with the Gwich'in in

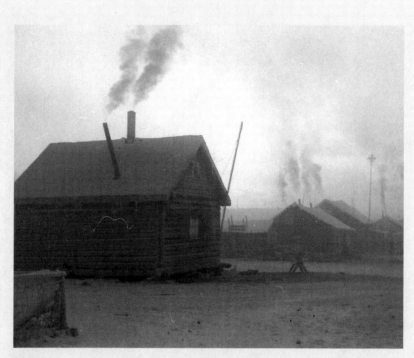

Stoves are at full blast on a cold January morning in the Gwich'in village.

1839, he found a large group of them camping at a place called Fish Trap Head on the Peel River, 160 kilometres from its mouth. The following year he established the first Bay Company post on the lower Peel, but very few Gwich'in came to trade because the goldfields were much closer to their hunting grounds and they could trade meat to the miners who were flocking to the rich goldfields around Dawson City. The Bay men soon discovered that their new fort's location was prone to flooding, so a few years later it was moved six kilometres downstream. It was planned at first to rebuild on the west bank of the river where the land was higher, but the Tetlit Gwich'in insisted that it should be built on the east side where they would have a clear view downriver in case an Eskimo raiding party should come when they were trading there. The new fort was first called Peel's River House after Sir Robert Peel, Britain's secretary of state, but it was later renamed in honour of Chief Factor Murdock McPherson. The Gwich'in established a village beside the fort in 1852.

The Fort McPherson Gwich'in (Tetlit Gwich'in) were closely related to the Vuntut Gwich'in of Old Crow in the Yukon and seemed to be more closely associated with them than with the geographically closer people of Arctic Red River (Tsiigehtchic Gwichya Gwich'in,) and the Aklavik people (Ehdi Tat Gwich'in). It is possible that religion had something to do with the association between villages as the people of both Old Crow and Fort McPherson were stalwart Anglicans and those of Arctic Red River Roman Catholic. On the other hand, the early explorers had noted that the people of Arctic Red River had a good trading relationship with the Eskimo, whom they referred to as "Huskies," and the Peel River people had very little to do with them, apart from sometimes trading at Fort McPherson or when either party was raiding the other. Because the Peel River people had traditionally lived at the upper reaches of the river, which is in the Ogilvie Mountains, and relied on caribou meat as did the people of Old Crow, it was possible that this was the basis for their affinity. Arctic Red River people subsisted mostly on fish, which the Mackenzie and Arctic Red rivers provided in abundance.

CHAPTER TWO

Before driving through Wrights Pass on the Dempster Highway, I stopped our truck and Muriel and I climbed out to stretch our legs. There was not a mosquito or blackfly to be seen or felt at this elevation, and for this we were very thankful. The lakes and rivers of the Peel Plateau shimmered in the August sun, and all around us lay a scene of incredible beauty and colour. This was a view that we had been unable to see when we had lived in Fort McPherson because in the summertime there had been no easy access to these hills and in the wintertime they were all covered with windswept snow, and whenever I had travelled over them with my dog team, I had been nestled deep in my fur-trimmed parka to keep my face out of the bitter wind. Now, as we looked out over the plateau, we could see the Peel River in the far distance with the faint outline of some houses on the riverbank. Fort McPherson! Our life there in the sixties had been exciting and fulfilling, though sometimes frightening, and many of our Gwich'in patients had become our friends. We had kept in contact with some of them over the years and we now looked forward to reliving our adventures with them.

Back in the truck, we descended from the high ground and drove the few kilometres past some small lakes to where the ferry *Abraham Francis* would provide a free crossing over the Peel. Because of heavy rains in the mountains at the head of the river, the water had risen in the past few days, and as we sat waiting for the ferry, we

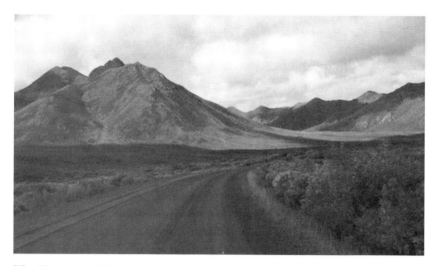

The Dempster Highway in August was in excellent shape.

watched forest debris floating past in the fast-moving, silty waters. A few small cabins sat in the thick undergrowth alongside the road but there was no sign of anyone living in them. When several monster trucks joined the ferry queue, I commented that they were just another sign of the progress that had been made in the North while we had been away. Or was it progress? we asked ourselves.

The *Abraham Francis* took us across the Peel to Eight Mile Point where a ramp had been built beside the ferry sheds, and it was up this ramp that the ferry would be hauled in October and where it would sit until the following May or June when the river ice broke up. Nearby, several long, wooden river boats were pulled up to the water's edge, their blunt prows sticking out over the muddy shore. A few old cabins were clustered around the terminal, and we realized that it had been to one of these cabins that Muriel and I had made our first trip by dogsled many years earlier and had learned that dogs knew how to fool a novice driver. After jogging behind the toboggan for most of the way back to the village in order to relieve "our poor tired dogs," they had spied another team ahead, and I had been unable to hold them back, even though I rode the sled with the brake dug deep into the snow!

Now, as we drove off the ferry and onto the gravel road, things began to look very familiar and yet different. It was not the only time we would think this on the trip because later as we met our old friends, most of whom we had not seen for a very long time, they, too, seemed the same except older and grayer, and some, like us, a little heavier. It was as if we had wakened after years of sleeping to find that time had flown by, leaving us feeling no different on the inside although a glance in a mirror confirmed that we were aging on the outside.

A sign at a junction in the road indicated that the branch to our left would take us to Fort McPherson while the road straight ahead continued east toward Tsiigehtchic, the small village that we had known as Arctic Red River. Both Muriel and I had travelled there many times long before this road had been built, sometimes in the relative comfort of an airplane but often by dog team, and I could well remember some exhilarating and some downright miserable trips with my dogs. A few days later we learned that the "traditional trail," the same dog team trail I had travelled, still existed, going from lake to lake over nearly forty portages to the last one, Islands Lake, close to Tsiigehtchic.

We turned off the Dempster Highway onto the road leading into the village of Fort McPherson, driving slowly, craning our heads to the left and right and remarking on the changes that were apparent. Dry roads had been built up off the permafrost, there was a gas station with real gas pumps, and prominent signs demanded that motorists "STOP" at intersections. But it was with delight that we saw that many roads had been named after Gwich'in people who had been the elders when we lived in the village, and that even the official buildings were named after elders. On the left side of the main road an imposing new two-storey building had been built on some high ground overlooking the Peel River. To us it looked like a small hotel, but there was a sign affixed to the front of the building: William Firth Health Centre.

William Firth had been the janitor and general handyman at

the old nursing station ever since it was built in the 1950s, and he had not retired until long after he had passed the mandatory retirement age of sixty-five. Many years earlier, he had been a manager at the Hudson's Bay Company store, following in his father's footsteps. Chief Factor John Firth had been a renowned figure in the North, very much respected and in many ways very much feared because these were the days when official lawmen were very few and far between in the Far North and the factor's word was law. John Firth had also acted as a lay dispenser of the medicines that were supplied by the Hudson's Bay Company, and he, like many other Bay managers across the North, had done his best to diagnose and treat the Native people who came for help. It seemed fitting, then, that William had migrated from the Bay first to spend years on a trapline, then to help build and care for the first medical building in Fort McPherson and finally to have the new health complex named after him.

After William's first wife died of tuberculosis, he married Mary Stewart with whom he raised another large family, so that now the Firth family was well represented in Fort McPherson, Aklavik and Inuvik. As William and Mary had lived just a few houses north of where the old nursing station had stood, they had become our good friends, helping us to understand the culture of the Gwich'in people and always ready to sort out the interwoven family relationships for us when we were doing medical investigations. After we had our two children, Helen and Stephen, Mary had become their babysitter when we were at work, and they spent most of their days in the little white wood-sided building with William or Mary. As Helen and Stephen's grandparents were thousands of kilometres away in England and because of the close relationship that developed between us, William became the children's *jijii* or grandfather, and Mary their *jijuu* or grandmother.

❄   ❄   ❄

I parked the truck and Muriel and I headed for the William Firth Health Centre to introduce ourselves and to ask permission to look around this wonderful new facility. The receptionist, Joanne Neyendo,

ALTHOUGH THE DRUM HAD BEEN THE instrument that the Gwich'in had traditionally used for ceremony and relaxation, after the fiddle was introduced to the North by either the French Canadian voyageurs or the men of the Hudson's Bay Company, many Gwich'in took up the fiddle. By the early 1940s there were a number of Gwich'in men who could play it well and they delighted in holding forth at community feasts and dances, playing for hours, sometimes alone and sometimes accompanied by a guitarist. William Firth learned to play the fiddle early in his life, and when there was no social reason to play, he would sit at home and play for his family. In time he became known as one of the best fiddle players in Fort McPherson, always in demand to play at feasts and dances.

However, when he was helping to construct the nursing station and everyone was rushing around trying to get the roof on before the weather turned bad, someone asked William to hurry and cut a piece of lumber. William grabbed the wood and placed it on the saw. Suddenly blood spurted everywhere. He was astonished to see it and wondered where it had come from. It was only when he saw that the tips of the fingers on his left hand were missing that he began to feel the pain.

Long after the surgery at the hospital in Aklavik—this happened before a hospital was built in Inuvik—and the healing process was well under way, William picked up his fiddle and tuned it. He tried a few notes and was disappointed to discover that he did not have any feeling in his fingertips. Though he tried to play several times, in the end he gave up in disgust, and despite a lot of encouragement from family and friends, he would not try again. He put his fiddle away so that he would be remembered as the excellent player he had been rather than one who had been a good player before he lost his touch.

welcomed us with a big smile and a hug and was soon reminding us that I had done some minor surgery on her little brother.

It had been late one afternoon in June 1964 when Mrs. Clara Neyendo had come into the clinic carrying her four-year-old boy, sat down on the clinic chair with her son snuggled up to her chest and handed me a scrunched-up piece of tissue paper. She explained that her son had been playing outside with a neighbour boy who had picked up the axe that was by the woodpile. Her little boy had put his right hand on the splitting block and the other boy had brought down the axe and cut off the end of her son's thumb. "I read that these days they can sew them back on," she said, "so I searched around until I found it and it's in that tissue!"

I opened the paper tissue and there was a tiny, very pale piece of thumb with a few wood chips adhering to it. I then examined the little boy's thumb—or more precisely what was left of it—and saw that it was cut off cleanly just below the end knuckle. I had seen a lot of plastic surgery done at the Camsell Hospital but I didn't think that any of the surgeons there could have reattached that tiny piece of digit. Besides, it was in the middle of breakup so I couldn't send the boy to Inuvik as no planes were flying. I told Clara that it would be impossible for me to reattach that minute bit of skin and bone, but I could sew up the end of the thumb so that it would look okay. He wouldn't have a thumb nail but I was sure he would soon learn to manage without it. She nodded in acceptance, though she was probably disappointed that her son would now have a very short thumb.

Meanwhile, the shock of the accident had caused the little boy to fall asleep, and when I injected some local anaesthetic into the thumb, all he did was flinch. His mother held his arm tight, looking away while I worked at loosening the skin around the little stump so that I could pull a flap over the end and sew it down with some fine catgut. I was nervous doing it, wondering how far I could go as a nurse. Was I overstepping the boundaries into "practicing medicine"? But what was the alternative?

45

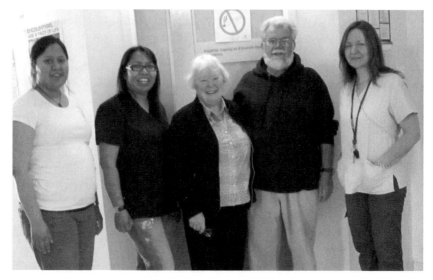

Jennifer, Janice and Carol welcomed us with big smiles.

I finished the last tiny stitch, cleaned the wound and put a dressing on it. Then I gave Clara some medicine that would keep the boy drowsy for the time being because I knew that his thumb was going to throb when the anaesthetic wore off. Within a week I was able to remove the stitches and found that the wound had healed well. That little boy carried on life just like any other little boy, adjusting to his shortened thumb and learning to write without any difficulty. In reminding us of her brother's accident, Joanne Neyendo finished her story by saying that it wasn't until many years later that he had some corrective surgery done, and I assumed that it was because the bone was pressing on the tight skin flap that I had made.

Carol McCormack, the nurse in charge of the new health centre, showed us around, and we were surprised to see that it was like a small hospital. She introduced us to two other registered nurses who were, to our utter delight, Gwich'in women from Fort McPherson—Jennifer and Janice Tetlichi, the granddaughters of the late John Tetlichi who had been chief when Muriel and I lived in Fort McPherson. Esther Blake, the home support worker, was also Gwich'in. They all welcomed us with big smiles.

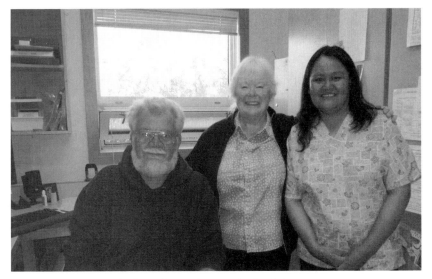

Muriel and I met Marlene Snowshoe at the health center.

Carol offered us one of the staff apartments on the second floor
of the building to stay in during our visit ("A *second* floor," we told
each other. "It's unbelievable!"), and as we went upstairs to the apartment, we were met by a young woman coming down. She looked
very familiar, and when Carol introduced us, a lump came into my
throat. Marlene was employed as the health centre's housekeeper,
and her mother, Maria Itsi, had been our housekeeper when we first
came to work in Fort McPherson. After Maria had been with us for
a year, she had married Neil Snowshoe and a short time later left
her job. Her first baby had died of hyaline membrane disease, and
then while Muriel was in Inuvik awaiting the arrival of our daughter
Helen, Maria had come to the nursing station in premature labour
with her second child. I had delivered her of a healthy baby girl
whom she named Marlene. Some time after that, Maria had accompanied her husband to his fishing camp, gone out in a canoe, fallen
overboard and drowned. Her body had been brought to our station
by the RCMP, and we had prepared and dressed her for burial, a very
difficult and upsetting task because of our close relationship during
her lifetime.

After Maria's death Muriel and I had seriously contemplated offering to adopt Marlene, as she was only slightly older than our daughter Helen and we felt a close attachment to her because of our association with Maria. It seemed unlikely that her father would be able to care for her since he spent much of his time out in the bush, and we didn't know who else would take her. But it was not to be.

When we met Marlene on the health centre stairs, she cried and gave us each a hug but for a while she could hardly speak. Meanwhile, her uncanny resemblance to her mother was quite unnerving for Muriel and me. Although she was as quiet and shy as her mother had been, she told us with a smile that she had wanted to meet us for a long time, then added that she now had a daughter whom she had named Maria.

❊   ❊   ❊

We were amazed at the size of the apartment that Carol had directed us to, which was as big as the total living quarters in our old nursing station. We were also awed at the relative opulence of the place—the high ceilings, a wide-screen television, a full kitchenette with fridge, stove and a full set of kitchen tools—things that we hadn't even dreamed of having in our old quarters. I looked at the telephone, and as though to acknowledge my glance, it rang and Muriel and I both jumped before realizing that it would be answered in the office.

When we had arrived in Fort McPherson in September 1963, there had been no phone in the nursing station, and we resisted having one installed because we thought that people would be calling us instead of coming to the nursing station where we had all the necessary supplies. So instead of phoning people, we sent our handyman, William Firth, with messages around the village, and for communication with Inuvik, 112 air kilometres north of Fort McPherson, we relied on the RCMP's single sideband radio.

By January 1964—just four months after our arrival in Fort McPherson—our work as nurses was becoming routine. We held treatment clinics every day during the week and on Wednesday evenings to treat coughs, colds and various aches and pains. We had also begun tuberculosis testing at the local Peter Warren Dease School. The children didn't particularly enjoy it because we were using a Heaf gun, which shot a small spiked plate onto the skin of the child's inner wrist where the testing material had been smeared. It didn't hurt but the spring-loaded gun made a metallic snap when I pulled the trigger and made the children jump.

Early in the month I made a trip to Arctic Red River, flying there in the regularly scheduled ski-equipped plane to see if anyone was ill and to give some of the children their vaccinations. I stayed at the RCMP corporal's house for the two nights I was there and went visiting the Gwich'in people house by house. While I was away, Muriel admitted one woman to the nursing station who was threatening to miscarry early in her pregnancy, then sent her home to rest, although Muriel knew this would be very difficult with two children and a hunter husband to look after in their small house. Almost immediately another woman arrived at the station in labour, and after Muriel had delivered the baby boy, mother and baby rested happily in our tiny maternity ward. By the time I arrived back from Arctic Red River, my wife and I had a lot to tell each other.

In late January a chinook raised the temperature dramatically from minus forty-five to a mere minus five degrees (Celsius), but we knew this respite would be short-lived and the biting cold would soon return. But there were no emergency calls where we had to brave the frozen elements in the middle of the night, and in between seeing a few patients in regular clinic hours, we started to compile the information that we needed for the monthly reports that had to be sent to our headquarters in Edmonton. Everything was quiet. Too quiet. We were about to be shaken out of our complacency.

At five-thirty one morning we were awakened by the clinic doorbell being rung very insistently. As I hurriedly pulled on some clothes, the doorbell continued its persistent ringing, jarring my nerves. "All right, all right, I'm coming, I'm coming," I said to no one in particular as though my message would get through to the buzzer.

Immediately, the clinic door opened and a very worried-looking woman rushed in, her parka pulled closely around her.

"I think I'm going to have my baby," she blurted, "but I'm not due yet!"

I made her comfortable in the small ward that Muriel and I had decided to keep for births, then went to tell Muriel that she had another maternity case to deal with. I knew that the patient's name was Mavis and I had her chart ready when Muriel came into the room and was able to confirm the dates Mavis had given me. Very carefully Muriel examined her and said that something was certainly happening, but when questioned, Mavis said that she hadn't felt the baby move much recently. Privately, Muriel expressed her concern to me. "I can't hear the fetal heart," she said then added, "Even if it is in a poor position, I should be able to hear something. Of course, the baby is premature but I think there's something very wrong. Will you go up to the RCMP office and call Inuvik for a plane?"

Dressing as fast as I could, I put on my winter clothes—long johns, wool pants, thick shirt, parka and moosehide mukluks—then went out into the cold. It was still night as far as I was concerned. The stars twinkled out of a clear sky and a frosty haze hung over the village, accentuated by the few street lamps on the main road. Living 160 kilometres inside the Arctic Circle gave us the rare experience of all light summer and all dark winter. Once the sun had set on the southern horizon on December 6, we didn't see it again until January 6 when it showed its rosy glow again for just a few minutes. But while we found this fascinating, the darkness was also very inconvenient when we needed to medevac a patient by plane to Inuvik General Hospital, over 120 kilometres to the North.

I walked hurriedly to the RCMP office and then, realizing that no one would be there yet, I went around to the corporal's house and banged on the door. Jim Hickling was used to being called out at all hours of the day or night, but like us he didn't particularly enjoy having someone pound on his door in the middle of the night, not knowing what sort of trouble he would be facing when he opened the door. But he ushered me into the house, and I explained our problem and asked if he would mind raising the Inuvik detachment on his radio.

After leading me into the office, he picked up his microphone from the desk in front of the radio and called Inuvik, identifying Fort McPherson detachment as the caller. There was no response. After several attempts with no reply, he tried calling Arctic Red River, then Fort Good Hope, but all he got back was the static sounds unique to such radios when what you really want to hear is a human voice responding. He examined all of his connections—power, aerial and mike—and everything seemed to be in order. He tried calling Inuvik again. Nothing.

"C'mon," he said, "I'll put the coffee pot on and we'll try again in a few minutes. This sometimes happens when there are freakish atmospheric conditions."

While we waited for the coffee to brew, we talked about family, friends and some of our plans both in this village and wherever the future would take us. Then we took the fresh coffee to the office and Jim tried calling Inuvik again, then Arctic Red River. "Sorry Keith, looks like the radio is down for awhile. I'll keep trying until I get a response from somewhere and let you know." I thanked him, finished my coffee and went back to the nursing station.

Muriel came out to the office, and I told her that for the moment we were on our own because we were unable to call Inuvik for a plane. "Well," she said. "Mavis still is not having any strong contractions. And so far she is not bleeding."

Mavis's husband, Tom, called by to see her, and we explained the situation. Muriel added that we wanted to keep Mavis as quiet as possible in the nursing station and asked him to tell her mother and others not to come to visit. We would let people know how she was faring through Tom.

The nursing station was quiet for most of the day, although someone did drop by to tell us that they thought there was an outbreak of chickenpox in the school hostel. We said we would check it out when possible. The matron there was a very capable woman and she would know what to do for her charges to make them as comfortable as possible.

Later that day I walked back up to the RCMP office to see if anything was happening, trying not to sound as though I were reminding them about our medical problem. Jim just shrugged and told me that both he and his partner had been trying their radio every fifteen minutes without any response. Again he promised to let me know just as soon as there was a response. I took this opportunity to cross the road to the hostel and within a few minutes was able to confirm that there was indeed chickenpox amongst the children. It was a relief to know that there were adequate supplies in the hostel dispensary that the matron could use to soothe the children's itchy skin.

It was just after four in the afternoon when Jim came into the clinic and beckoned Muriel and me into our office. He asked how our patient was doing and we explained that there was virtually no change. Muriel had checked and double-checked for the fetal heartbeat and then had me check, using the large fetal stethoscope. No movement and no heartbeat.

Then Jim told us that he had finally made contact by radio. "Fort Good Hope had heard us calling for some time, but we couldn't hear them so they passed a message to Arctic Red River, and just before four they reached us and asked what our problem was. Anyway, we passed on your message and they relayed it to Inuvik and then told us that a plane will be here in about an hour. We still haven't been able to talk directly to Inuvik ourselves, but it looks as though the weather's slowly clearing up." He started for the door then stopped. "I've got to get some lights down on the runway so Freddy Carmichael can land. Have you got some spare toilet rolls we can use?" Seeing our raised eyebrows, he smiled and told us that he soaked the rolls in kerosene and then, when the plane's lights could be seen in the distance, they set the rolls alight to provide long-lasting runway lights alongside the improvised airstrip. I found half a case of toilet rolls for him and thanked him for his help.

"Anytime," he said, "but I hope not too often before breakfast! I'll be back with the truck to take Mavis down when the plane is close."

We wrapped Mavis in blankets and placed her on a stretcher while we waited for the sound of the small plane, but before it came, we heard the truck outside and a moment later Jim was standing in the door again. "Let's go!" he called, "I just saw the plane's lights over to the north, and the men are down there lighting our flares."

By the time we reached the airstrip, Freddy Carmichael's small plane was touching down between the flickering and smoking runway "lights," and I can remember hoping that we wouldn't have to do this too often or we would be running short of a valuable and essential commodity before next summer when the barge came in again!

Dr. Joseph Cramer, a well-respected doctor—and the only one stationed at the Inuvik General Hospital at that time—jumped out of the plane and we hurriedly took him aside and told him about Mavis' condition. Without any fuss he listened, thanked us and organized Mavis in the plane where she had been placed by helpful hands. Within minutes the plane was on its way back to Inuvik, leaving Muriel and I greatly relieved. We accepted a ride back to the nursing station where as usual we set to work cleaning up to be ready for the next patient. By nine-thirty in the evening we were both so tired that we went to bed, hoping for a quiet night.

At mid-morning the next day Jim called by to tell us that communications were back to normal and Dr. Cramer had passed a message through the Inuvik detachment that Mavis's baby had been born dead, something we had feared was a strong possibility. Jim had already been to see Tom to tell him this sad news, and we were thankful that we were spared this. It was unfortunate that Mavis was now all alone in Inuvik because we could imagine her grief at losing her baby and not having her husband or other family members there to console her.

❄   ❄   ❄

The following day was more seasonable, clear and cold with

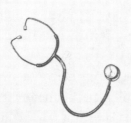

MANY OF THE DOCTORS WHO ACCEPTED positions in the North only stayed for short periods of time, but Dr. Joseph E. Cramer provided medical services in Inuvik for four years in all during the mid-sixties. He was born in Drumheller, Alberta, in 1928 and graduated in medicine from the University of Alberta in 1958. He interned at the Edmonton General and did post-graduate training at St. Joseph's Hospital in Flint, Michigan, followed by a residence in surgery at the Edmonton General Hospital. He served as the primary medical doctor in Inuvik from early 1963 to October 1964 when he began practicing in northern Alberta, although he returned to Inuvik many times to provide medical services until 1967. He and his wife, Mary Anne, died on October 31, 1970, when the light plane he was piloting crashed near High River, Alberta. He was forty-two.

the thermometer hovering around minus thirty-eight degrees (C), which didn't seem too extreme for the last day of January. Muriel donned her parka and braved the outdoors so that she could make a few home visits to frail elders whom we liked to keep an eye on during the winter months, and I tried to catch up on our reports and requisitions. That evening we held a first aid class for the fire department, after which we called in at the home of our teacher friends, Mike and Bett Wiggins, who were holding a square dance party. After the tensions of the previous day it was relaxing to literally kick up our heels with a houseful of people, but after working up a sweat dancing, it was a shock to step outside at two in the morning and feel the frost attacking our perspiring brows. However, it was Saturday and we assumed that we could lie in bed for a bit longer in the morning.

The clinic doorbell rang little more than two and a

half hours later. More bleary-eyed than usual, I went to the door to find an apologetic young man named Andy, who implored me to come and see his wife in their house, which was just a few minutes walk from the nursing station. He said that she had wakened a short time earlier and found that she was bleeding heavily. Anticipating that we would be admitting his wife to the nursing station, I gave him our portable stretcher and told him I would be following him just as soon as I could get dressed. I told Muriel what was happening and she prepared a bed while I bundled up and went down to the house.

Fifteen minutes later I entered the small clapboard house where Mary and Andy lived and immediately shucked off my parka as the heat from their roaring wood stove was blasting out. Mary lay on the low wooden bed and gave me a weak smile. She said that she was about three months pregnant and a casual observation showed that she was indeed bleeding heavily. "Let's get her to the station right away," I said and unfolded the stretcher. We lifted her, using the sleeping bag she was in, and placed her on the stretcher. With Andy at the rear of the stretcher and me in front, we left the house, only pausing while Andy closed the door behind him.

Muriel was ready for us. We laid Mary on the bed and Andy left the room as Muriel prepared to examine her. I tried to take her blood pressure but it was so low that it was difficult to get a reading. Muriel cleaned Mary up and soon determined that she had spontaneously aborted but that it was incomplete, meaning that there was still some tissue in the womb, and this was causing the bleeding to continue. We lifted the foot of the bed and propped it on a chair so that Mary's head was much lower than her body, then we started an intravenous infusion of 5 percent Dextrose to try to replace some of the fluid that had been lost with the hemorrhage.

This time my visit to the RCMP office produced better results. Jim received an answer from Inuvik almost immediately and within a very short time I had given the doctor an outline of the problem. He promised to send a plane and said he would try to find an off-duty nurse from the hospital who would act as the patient's escort.

The plane had arrived by mid-morning and we saw Mary off to the hospital with a nurse escort. Some time later we heard that Mary was doing fine after having surgery and a D&C and could be expected home again within the week. Meanwhile, Muriel and I had returned to the nursing station to clean up. We put the sheets and other soiled linen into the washing sink to soak and await our housekeeper's return on Monday when she would do our regular daily cleaning. When we finally sat down in the kitchen with cups of coffee, I commented, "This has been quite a busy few days, hasn't it?"

"Yes," Muriel said. "I wonder what will happen next?"

CHAPTER THREE

IN MID-1964, AS THE RESULT OF a new government policy
to bring the North into communication with the rest of the
country, Canada National Communications (CNT) installed
a microwave tower in the Fort McPherson community and phones
in all the government offices, and we gave in at last and had one
installed in the nursing station. After that, we didn't get quite as
much exercise because we could now call the various agencies to
make enquiries or to advise them of a problem, and because many of
the townspeople also got phones at this time, we rarely had to send
William on some midnight mission to alert a family of an accident.
But the best part about having a phone was that we were now able
to call the Inuvik General Hospital for advice, although this rarely
happened because we had already become so used to managing on
our own. However, when there was a real emergency, it certainly
was less stressful to talk directly to a doctor or to call for a medevac
plane ourselves. Since Muriel and I were responsible for the health
of all the residents of the village and we found ourselves caring for
people from birth up to and even after death, having easy access to
a phone and a plane did make us breathe easier.

But the phones were far from trouble-free. Much of the time
the line was almost unusable because of the static, and placing a
long distance call was extremely complicated. I remember trying to
call Muriel after I had been delayed by weather at a small Eskimo

settlement at Cape Parry in the Beaufort Sea where I had gone to immunize some children and investigate possible dietary problems in the community. My phone call had first to be relayed down to Pyramus in New Jersey because I was calling from a Distant Early Warning (DEW) site run mostly by the American army. It was then relayed back up to Canada through Edmonton and then Inuvik, but as the microwave was not functioning that day, the message did not get through until I had arrived home some days later. After that experience we only called out of the settlement when we really had to. Meanwhile, the RCMP continued to use their single sideband radio, which was much better than the CNT line 95 percent of the time.

However, as we had feared, there were a few people in Fort McPherson who took advantage of the fact that we now had a phone and would call to tell us that someone—never the individual who was calling—was really sick and ask if we would come right away. So one of us would drop what we were doing and rush up to the house, only to be met at the door by an individual who had run out of his pills and wanted us to go and get some for him.

I was quite annoyed at one woman who had me over a barrel with her demand that I come to her house and see her little girl who had swallowed some toothache drops. I told her that she should bring the little girl down to the nursing station where we had the equipment and any supplies we might need right at hand.

"No, you come up here," she said. "It's your job to take care of the people!" and she hung up.

I was in a quandary. On one hand, the amount of toothache drops in the bottles we dispensed was minimal, and as the major ingredient was cloves, there should be no harm, and the responsibility lay with the mother. On the other hand, what if the little girl was really ill because of both ingesting *and* inhaling the drops? Or what if she had taken something else that was really toxic and hadn't told her belligerent mother?

There was no Social Services person in the village to whom I could complain, so in order to have peace of mind, I went to the house. The child was quietly playing in a corner of the cabin and showing no signs of discomfort. She looked up at me and smiled, so I tore a strip off the woman who had called and told her if there was a next time she would have to call the Indian agent first and he would come with me to investigate. At the same time I knew that if there was a next time I would still respond because I would be worried about her child.

Ah, phones! We couldn't do with them and soon found that we couldn't do without them, and like lots of things that were happening in Fort McPherson, it was going to take time for people to learn how and when to use them.

Of all the medical emergencies that we had to deal with, those that involved mothers and babies were the most common and the most alarming, as well as the ones that most often required the use of the telephone. At such times concentration and speed were necessary, and as maternal and child health was Muriel's specialty, she often bemoaned the lack of supplies in the nursing station. We did not have an incubator, so when a premature birth occurred, while Muriel was concentrating on the birth and the baby, I would be constructing a makeshift incubator out of our newborn crib, hot water bottles and oxygen. The babies gave us sleepless nights at times and our ears were always attuned to them, interpreting their cries, but in the six years that we were in Fort McPherson we only lost one newborn and that was because he had hyaline membrane disease, a lung problem of premature babies.

Muriel excelled in diagnosing problems associated with pregnancy. She obviously enjoyed this part of the nursing program and over the years delivered lots of babies. When we visited Fort McPherson in later years it was always a surprise when someone would casually remark, "You delivered my Mitch" or some other name that usually meant nothing to us because when they were delivered they were simply "newborn male (or female)."

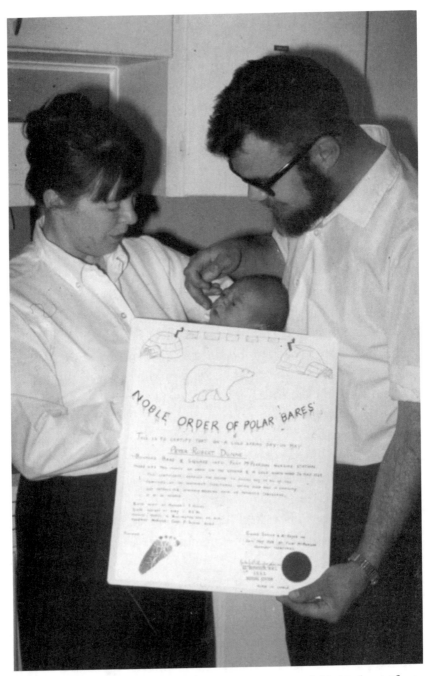

Noble order of polar bares: baby Frank Dunn poses with his birth certificate
a la Fort McPherson. FRANK DUNN PHOTO.

When everything went well at a delivery, it was a joy, with proud parents, grandparents and other kin. When things went awry, it was panic stations. I once asked Muriel why babies always seemed to be born late at night or very early in the morning, because we rarely had daytime deliveries. We decided that maybe it was that boost in a woman's energy level just prior to a birth that made her scoot around at home during the day and set her up for a late delivery!

Early one evening in 1965 Bertha Martin came to the nursing station in labour. She was a good-looking, slightly built Gwich'in woman, who had a quiet smile and an infectious laugh. She kept her small clapboard house spotless, and her three children and her husband, James, were all well cared for. He had a steady job in the village and was known to be a sober and caring man.

Muriel had seen her regularly throughout her pregnancy and everything seemed to be progressing satisfactorily, except that ideally Bertha should have gone to Inuvik for delivery as she was classed as a multipara. The policy was that all first and fourth babies should be born in hospital because they were at a higher risk.

Around ten-thirty that night a baby's loud cry came from the birthing room as he entered the cool cruel world. Afterwards, with his umbilical cord tied and cut, he was placed on his mother's chest to be admired. Then Muriel put the baby in a preheated crib and turned her attention back to Bertha. It was at about this point that I went to see what was happening, and Muriel said that the placenta (the afterbirth) had not yet delivered, and Bertha was bleeding quite heavily. Muriel had given Bertha an injection of ergometrine, which is used to assist the uterus to contract and, in this case, expel the placenta and stop any bleeding, but Bertha's pulse rate was increasing and she continued to bleed. Muriel was concerned that she had done something wrong because this was the first time that this had happened and she realized that it was very serious.

While I prepared a dextrose-saline intravenous drip for Bertha and started it, Muriel spoke to the doctor in Inuvik, explaining that the patient had a retained placenta and was bleeding heavily and we did not have any blood or even plasma to give, which was what Bertha needed. When she hung up the phone, she turned with relief to tell me that two doctors were going to try and fly in with Freddy Carmichael, the owner and pilot of Reindeer Air Services, and would be arriving in just over an hour. The doctor had directed Muriel to elevate the foot of the bed and then, if nothing happened, to give another shot of ergometrine. I lifted the foot of the bed and Muriel slid a chair under the frame, then we increased the flow of the drip.

While Muriel continued to monitor Bertha's vital signs, I pushed the buzzer that was connected to the Firths' house a short distance away to alert William that we had an emergency. When he appeared a few minutes later, we dispatched him to the Martins' house, where there wasn't a phone, to let James know that he was the father of another boy and that his wife was having some problems and he should come down to the nursing station. Next I phoned the RCMP and they went into high gear to get the airstrip on the sandbar lit up, using the tried and true method of lighted kerosene-soaked toilet rolls.

We moved the baby in his crib to the adjoining ward, then while Muriel attended to Bertha, I put up another IV bottle with saline and, on the advice of the doctors, started a second IV in Bertha's other arm but kept it at a slow rate. Bertha was very quiet, her face pale and her pulse rate fast but not very strong. James came in and sat holding his wife's hand, not saying a word, but his concern showed on his face as he watched us working around her. At last we heard Freddy's plane fly overhead with a roar to alert us to his arrival, but we knew that both the corporal and the constable were down on the sandbar waiting to bring the doctors up.

Throwing their coats off as they came in, doctors Wright and McNay donned the gowns that we had prepared for them and then rubber gloves. I was relieved to see that they had brought several bottles of plasma and one was immediately attached to the second IV that I had prepared. Doctor Wright told me they were going to have to do a manual removal of the placenta and asked me to make

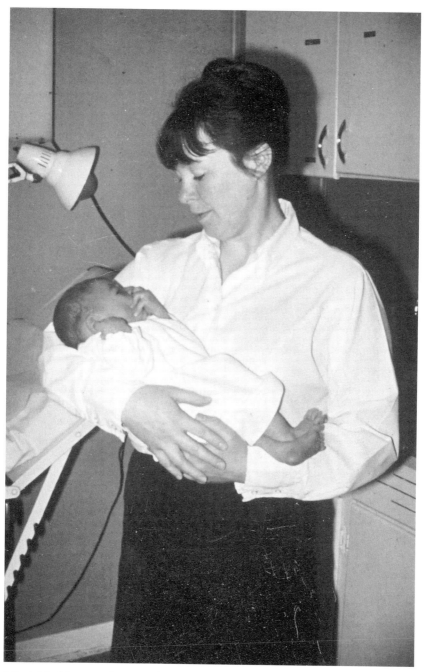

Muriel holds a newborn at the clinic. FRANK DUNN PHOTO.

sure that there was no open flame anywhere because they had to use ether as an anaesthetic, and it is a very volatile liquid.

The procedure lasted only a few minutes, but Bertha was only half-anaesthetized and we could hear her groans. Then Dr. McNay gave her another injection and packed the area, but as he was now worried about secondary shock from loss of blood, he also put up another bottle of plasma. Then we watched and waited. Bertha was nauseated from the ether, but we were all relieved when she opened her eyes and began to look more alert. The doctor explained what they had done and that they were now going to wait awhile to make sure that she had stopped bleeding.

James came back into the room to sit by Bertha, and after checking the baby, Muriel and I headed for the kitchen. There we joined Freddy Carmichael and the two Mounties who had brought the doctors up in their truck, then gone back to collect Freddy because no one knew how long the plane would have to wait. We all stood around drinking coffee, waiting to see how things were going to turn out.

Dawn was breaking when the decision was made to take Bertha to Inuvik where she could have a blood transfusion and possibly more surgical treatment if it was necessary. One of the Mounties took Freddy down to the plane to warm it up while we wrapped Bertha warmly and put her on a stretcher. Dr. Wright carried the baby who was going to accompany his mom to the hospital. When the Mountie returned with the truck, Bertha was carried out and taken down to the plane, and when everyone was on board, Freddy took off.

The nursing station looked like a tornado had been through it. We piled stacks of soiled linens in the utility room, glad that our housekeeper, Rachel Stuart, would soon be along to start her chores.

William came in after we had eaten a late breakfast. His job was to make sure that the placenta was burned up completely so that ravens or loose dogs did not get at it. He told us that the old people were very particular about this, as there was some belief about the spiritual properties of the placenta.

It was hard for Muriel and me to relax after all the activity and stress, and while we cleaned up the clinic and maternity room, we discussed the past evening's events. It was cold comfort to know that if this had happened not too many years earlier, Bertha would have died—as we knew that she had come perilously close to doing that night. If it hadn't been for the willingness of Freddy and the two doctors to risk their lives flying in the dark, there could have been a tragedy.

❄   ❄   ❄

In the years after the phone was installed in the nursing station, it jarred us from slumber into adrenaline-fed action many, many times. I remember one of those occasions in particular when the phone rang while we were fast asleep. I rolled over in bed and glanced at the bedside clock. Four o'clock! I struggled out of bed and staggered into the sitting room to answer the persistently ringing phone.

"Sorry to bother you, Keith, but Carolyn is having a problem. She's only thirty-six weeks and she has started to bleed."

My mind started to clear as I recognized the deep voice of Ben, the village game warden, and I knew that he would not have called without good reason. I asked him if his wife was having contractions but he said that he didn't think so—not real contractions, just some cramps. I told him that I would get Muriel to check her out, and he said that he would be able to bring Carolyn down to the nursing station in his truck. I hung up the phone and went to wake Muriel but found her already dressing.

"I heard you talking to Ben and I could tell by the conversation that you would be calling me in a minute!"

We both dressed and went into the kitchen where I cranked up the oil stove. It always surprised me how quickly I could come awake and be so business-like when there was a medical emergency. Most mornings in the wintertime I would get out of bed and move around slowly, sipping coffee as my mind caught up with the rest of my body. Nothing like a shot of adrenaline to get me activated!

"What's the temperature like this morning?" Muriel asked as she pulled on a sweater. "It sure feels chilly and the oil furnace has been chugging away for ages."

I pulled back the curtain and peered at the thermometer fastened outside the window. "It's minus forty-two degrees at the moment, but I don't think there's any wind."

Very shortly we heard a truck drive by the entrance to our living quarters and pull up in front of the clinic. We had the door open even as Ben was helping his wife up the steps. "Come right into the clinic room," Muriel told Carolyn, who, although pale and concerned, mumbled an apology for disturbing us at such an early hour. "I'm sure that you didn't plan this," Muriel said with a smile. She shut the clinic door behind them.

"C'mon, Ben," I said. "Let's go and put the coffee on. They might be a while yet." And we walked down the short corridor to the station's kitchen.

But before the coffee had finished brewing, Muriel opened the clinic door. "Keith!" she called. When I joined her in the office, she said, "I can't be positive but I think that Carolyn has a placenta previa and we are going to have to get her to hospital."

This is a serious medical problem and we both knew it could result in the death of both mother and child if we could not arrange a Caesarian section. I glanced out the window and thought about the temperature. "How long do you think we can wait?"

"We can't. We will have to call for a medevac right away, and if they can't come, you'd better get ready to do a Caesar!"

"Okay, I get the picture."

Muriel made Carolyn comfortable on one of the ward beds and warned her not to try to get up or move around. I relayed the problem to Ben, and he went home to collect some clothes and personal items for his wife. As soon as he left the nursing station, I picked up the phone and dialed the Inuvik hospital.

By this time Dr. Joe Cramer had returned south, and we were not sure who we would reach, if anyone, but this was a good day, and it did not take Dr. Al Aubrey more than a few minutes to reach the phone. I explained our concern and after a few perfunctory questions he said that he would phone Freddy Carmichael and call us back when a flight time was arranged. To my relief he also said that he would come with Freddy and escort the patient back to Inuvik; this meant he would take over the responsibility, although Muriel and I would be ready to assist with whatever treatment was necessary. It was very comforting to know that the doctors always took our word when we told them our diagnosis of a particular patient, and though they would ask a few appropriate questions, they were always willing to listen to our plea for help.

Muriel and I had trained as nurses in Halifax, England, at a general hospital where we were expected to know everything about our patients, and when we did ward rounds with the doctors, we had to give the details of the patient, then the diagnosis, the differential diagnosis, the treatment regimen that the patient was on, all the possible side effects of the treatment and, last of all, the prognosis. All of this prepared us for nursing in remote areas of the world where a doctor may or may not be available. Muriel, a gold medal recipient, had also trained as a midwife and a district midwife in the north of England where she had witnessed almost every complication of childbirth. She had also taught me the finer points of delivering a baby, but I was happy to leave that particular aspect of nursing in her capable hands.

My own expertise as a graduate nurse had been mainly on the surgical ward and in the operating room where I had been given the opportunity to assist at many of the surgical procedures. The surgeons had been very instructive—"Feel the tissue, Keith, but gently!"—and they would point out the various organs in the abdominal cavity, then as we began to finish up, I would be handed forceps and told to start suturing the incision. I was confident that if ever I had to remove an appendix, I could do it, but I would want someone else to give the anaesthetic, first to the patient then save some for me!

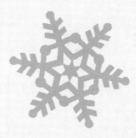

FOR COMMUNICATION WITH PEOPLE OUT IN the bush, Radio Station CHAK, launched in 1960 as part of the CBC's Northern Radio Service, was the lifeline for the communities. From Cape Parry and Paulatuk on the coast to Norman Wells and Fort Wrigley to the south, everyone listened to the station and, apart from the fact that there was no other station to listen to, it was the station that bonded northerners together. At lunchtime, suppertime and a trapper's bedtime, for the few minutes that the program "Neighbourly News and Messages" was on the air, silence reigned across the Delta.

I had used the program to let people know of emergencies regarding their families. I had also used it to send the message to the community as a whole that our first child had been born. In the Gwich'in tradition I said the baby was a "shoemaker," because it was the women in Fort McPherson who made all the moccasins and mukluks. The Gwich'in immediately knew that we had a baby girl. Later, when our first son Stephen was born, I was able to send another message saying that Muriel had delivered "a young trapper."

As is usual with community radio, the announcers became household names, but a couple in particular were very familiar to us. Ernest Firth, who had a very smooth and relaxed radio voice, was William Firth's son, as was Walter Firth, who started out in radio and later piloted his own plane around his huge riding in his capacity as the federal representative for the Northwest Territories. Nellie Cournoyea, who was born in Aklavik of Norwegian and Inupiaq heritage, was also an announcer and station manager for CHAK. On one mainliner trip from Yellowknife to Inuvik, when a

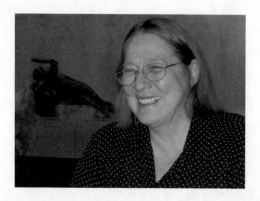

Nellie Cournoyea served as the first female premier of the Northwest Territories from 1991 to 1995. PHOTOGRAPH COURTESY OF BARTLETT-LEROSE PRODUCTIONS.

crowd of us were returning from a conference on the upcoming Territorial Centennial, she and Bob McCleverty, one of the supervisors from Fleming Hall, kept us amused by reading comics aloud to us, using super-refined CBC voices. Nellie Cournoyea became a successful politician and the first female premier of the Northwest Territories (1991 to 1995).

In later years Fort McPherson had its own local radio station, staffed by volunteers. Its programs were designed for the Gwich'in people, and some were delivered in Tukudh, the local language. There were health broadcasts, jigging music and local news and messages. One of the popular voices was that of Neil Colin, and I had a good laugh when I found out that Neil, who is never at a loss for words and who owns a cabin at the Mouth of the Peel River, is jokingly called "The Mouth of the Peel."

The phone rang and the doctor told Muriel that he was at the plane base ready to take off and should be arriving in about an hour. By this time Ben had returned to the nursing station with a bag of clothes and personal effects for his wife, and when he overheard Muriel repeat what Dr. Aubrey had said, he headed out to warm up his truck again. The sky was overcast and grey. The temperature was still minus forty degrees and everything outside was stiff with the cold so even with the truck's heater going full blast, it would still be cold inside the truck.

"The doctor will want to examine Carolyn before he takes her on the plane!" I shouted to him as he went down the steps. "You'll need to bring him up here first and that will speed things up." He waved and with the tires squeaking on the frigid snow he drove out of the yard and headed down to the snow-covered landing strip.

Some months earlier a section of the sandbar on the near side of the Peel River had been cleared of debris and a number of small spruce trees had been placed along each side of what was now a runway big enough for the single Otter that Pacific Western Airways used for their scheduled stop at Fort McPherson. We knew that Freddy Carmichael's small Cessna 185 would have no difficulty landing and taking off.

The sky was still grey when we heard the sound of the small plane buzzing the village to alert us to Freddy's arrival, and peering out of the window into the Arctic morning, I could make out two vehicles down at the strip, Ben's at one end and I guessed the one at the other end would be the RCMP truck. The plane's intensely bright landing lights had been switched on and I watched as the Cessna touched down gently in a flurry of snow.

Ten minutes later Ben's truck squeaked into the yard again and I heard truck doors slamming. Ben left the engine running as Dr. Aubrey came into the station, taking off his parka even as he shook our hands and laughingly asked why it was always so cold when we called him out! We offered him a cup of fresh coffee, which he drank while he perused Carolyn's file, then he and Muriel went into the small ward where Carolyn lay. Within minutes they came out and Dr. Aubrey confirmed Muriel's diagnosis, explained the situation to Ben who just nodded, then Ben came with me to transfer his wife onto the stretcher that we had already prepared with several warm blankets.

The ride down to the airstrip was most uncomfortable for Carolyn because she was on a stretcher in the cold back of the pickup while Ben sat in the warm interior of the truck to drive, a fact that he sheepishly admitted he had not thought about. Muriel and I squatted in the freezing cold on either side of Carolyn to keep the stretcher as still as possible, and we were all thankful when we finally arrived at the plane. Freddy had put a canvas cover over the plane's engine to try to retain some heat, and now he took the cover off and stowed it in the back of the small plane. Then between us we angled the stretcher this way and that way until finally we could place it on the floor of the Cessna. After Dr. Aubrey had climbed aboard, Freddy swung up into his seat and fastened his seat belt. We watched as he shut the door firmly and, after doing his pre-flight check, start the engine and wave goodbye. For a moment a cloud of blue smoke surrounded us and the wind created by the props made us turn our backs. Then with a roar the plane was hurtling down the runway and up into the still dusky sky.

Ben drove us home, and as he left us at the clinic door, he told us that as soon as he had contacted his office in Inuvik he would take the scheduled Pacific Western Airways flight to Inuvik. We tidied up the clinic room and remade the bed that Carolyn had used, then we went into the kitchen and relaxed with a cup of coffee. "I guess it's no good going back to bed now, is it?" I said. "It's almost time to start the treatment clinic." So we made breakfast and ate our cereal and wondered what the new day would bring.

It was mid-afternoon before the telephone rang and I heard Dr. Aubrey's voice. "Well, we did a C-section on Carolyn and she now has a six-pound boy! Both are doing well and Ben arrived in time to see her just as she came out of the OR." We thanked him for the news and settled down over our mid-afternoon coffee break to talk about all the "what ifs" that had been involved. What if the weather had been bad? What if there had been no doctor available? What would have happened only a few years earlier when there was no professional help available? What would the repercussions have been if all else had failed and the only way to avoid a dead mother and baby had been for me to…? I shuddered at the thought. Although we had sometimes thought how romantic it would have been to have lived a hundred years earlier, at times like this we were glad to have the technology that the world gave to us now, even though the availability of this technology was very limited in Canada's North.

Having made a correct diagnosis on such a complicated maternity case was very encouraging for Muriel, especially since there are not too many cases like this even in large maternity hospitals. But less than a week after we sent Carolyn out to Inuvik, another very pregnant woman came in with the same symptoms. This woman had been to see us many times in the past few months, usually complaining of problems that she was sure would necessitate her having to go to Inuvik, but after examining her, Muriel and I decided that the diagnosis was "thirst"—she and her husband were concocting reasons for her to go to Inuvik because that's where the liquor store was located. So now the first thing we thought was that this was another attempt to fool us.

But after Muriel had carefully examined her, she discussed the situation with me. "The doctor is not going to believe this," she said despairingly. "There is no way that we could be having another case the same as Carolyn's, but I am sure that it is, and in spite of all the fluff that she has given us in the past, I really do think that she has a placenta previa, which is serious."

Years earlier when Muriel was having her final midwifery exam, she had defended a diagnosis she had made and felt that the examiner was trying to make her uncertain when he kept asking her, "Are you sure?" Muriel had quietly reviewed all of her findings and still came up with the same diagnosis—which proved to be correct.

72

I picked up the phone and dialed the hospital and then handed the phone to Muriel and she explained her findings. After a few minutes I heard her say, "Yes, I find it hard to believe, too, but I have gone over everything again and again, and it just can't be anything else." She listened for a few moments and then said, "Thank you. We'll have everything ready when you get here."

We made arrangements to have the patient taken to the airstrip on a stretcher, watched the plane land and within minutes the patient was transferred from the truck to the plane and the doctor took charge. Back at the nursing station we waited for a phone call from the hospital, hoping that the mother and baby would be okay but also secretly hoping also that in spite of the odds Muriel's diagnosis had been correct.

The phone rang, and even though we were expecting it, the jangling machine made us jump. "Go ahead," I said to Muriel, indicating the phone. She picked it up and a smile spread over her face as Dr. Aubrey confirmed her diagnosis and she heard that the mother had delivered a healthy baby boy by Caesarian section. As Muriel sank into her armchair with a satisfied look on her face, she said, "I don't care what the statistics say, I have seen enough of those kinds of cases for my lifetime."

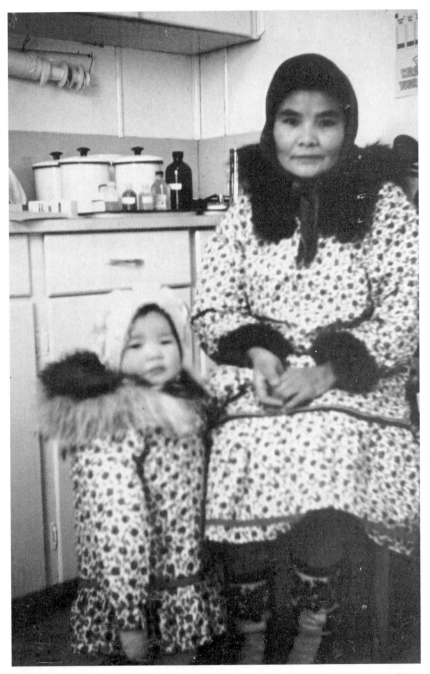

Elizabeth Mitchell stands with young daughter Mary at the clinic in Fort McPherson, 1964.

CHAPTER FOUR

W HEN WE RETURNED TO FORT MCPHERSON in 2009, it was rather embarrassing to meet people on the street who recognized us, even though we had changed a lot, while over the years we had forgotten their names. We also knew that some of the older people had lost their partners, those in our age group had become, like us, grandparents and the children we had known had become men and women. Obviously, we needed to be brought up to date on who was who.

There is usually at least one person in any community you can rely on to give you straight answers, and in Fort McPherson that person was Mary Teya, who now lived next door to the William Firth Health Centre. We had been in contact with her on an irregular basis for many years, and several years before our 2009 visit, when I had been working for a First Nations band in British Columbia, I had flown to Inuvik on business and persuaded the pilot to land in Fort McPherson as it was not far out of our way. We had put down at the new airport and hitched a ride to Mary's house, where we were welcomed with open arms. It was as if I had seen her only days earlier. She had never met the pilot who was with me, but she offered us breakfast and coffee and we sat and talked about old times. A kind and caring person, she took everything in her stride and never seemed to get into a flap.

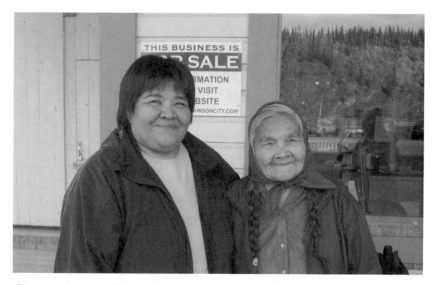

Changes happen! Forty-five years later: Mary Teya and her mother Elizabeth in Dawson City, 2009.

Now, in answer to our knock, she greeted us at the door with a big smile and a hug, and soon we were sitting down in her kitchen as though it was a regular occurrence. It made us feel quite strange because this was the same scene that had occurred forty years earlier, in our last year in Fort McPherson, when Mary had taken over the job of housekeeper from Rachel Stuart, and we had all sat around the kitchen table in the nursing station many times. Now here we were in Mary's kitchen again and it wasn't long before we were enjoying some fresh bannock and drinking tea just like the old days!

Mary had quite a resume, having worked first at the nursing station as housekeeper and later as a health worker; she had been on the band council and acted as the band chief, and later she was ordained as a minister in the Anglican Church. In fact, on this trip, when we had first driven into the village and gone to her house, we were told that she was away, having been called to Tuktoyaktuk to perform a marriage ceremony, but she was expected back later in the day. But even with all of this in her background, she remained a very humble person.

Her husband, William Teya, a rather shy and smiling man, had also been our friend and had taken me on my first dog team trip to Arctic Red River. He had been one of the group who made a dog team trip with me to Dawson City in 1970 as part of the Northwest Territories Centennial "Lost Patrol" re-enactment. I had last seen him in 1995 when we both attended the RCMP Ball in Dawson City prior to the Mounties' re-enactment of the old patrol to Fort McPherson. However, in 2008 William disappeared while trying to cross the Peel River from the Teyas' cabin on the west side of the river and is presumed to have drowned. Now as Mary sat in her kitchen, she was surrounded by walls covered with photographs of her family, and in a prominent position was a large photo of William. She spoke calmly and honestly about him, having come to terms with her loss, and we were able to reminisce without any sadness.

"Keith," she said suddenly, "do you remember that trip you made up the river with Don Wootten and Peter Thompson?" Don was the Anglican minister and Peter a church catechist, and they had travelled with me up to Three Cabin Creek by dogsled. "Sarah, she still talks about those teeth you fixed for her up there," Mary said, smiling. "It sure was a pity about Brian, though."

It had been late spring, an appropriate time to plan a visit to the camps up the Peel River, to make sure that everyone was healthy before the imminent ice breakup when no one would be able to move either on the river or over land. Earlier that spring I had travelled with Peter and Don on an aborted trip up Vittrekwa Creek when we had been turned back by bitterly cold weather and expanses of water on top of the creek ice and finally by my succumbing to a bout of diarrhea. This time we were going as far south as Three Cabin Creek, which was about thirty-five kilometres on the Peel River ice.

Travelling in a convoy, we reached Eight Mile Point where Peter Vittrekwa was camping in his small cabin, and seeing smoke coming from the chimney, we pulled off the river to visit him and give our dogs a short rest. We enjoyed tea and bannock with Peter and his wife and discussed their trapping and their health, and they told us that they planned to come to town as soon as the ice had cleared off the river. Out on the river again we moved slowly along the trail, neither the dogs nor ourselves being in a hurry. Peter Thompson would often tell us that both he and his dogs were old and moved slowly. "No use to hurry!" he would say, a broad smile creasing his round face.

I had heard that the people in Old Crow, the nearest Gwich'in village to the west, had said that the people of Fort McPherson had lost their traditional behaviour protocols, but there continued to be several families who seemed to be socially a cut above many of the others in the way they treated each other, the elders and even people from Outside. Peter Thomspson was one of those who continued to embody the old Gwich'in character of politeness and proper protocol, which to a lot of modern young people seemed a bit old-fashioned. When he met Muriel on the street, he would touch his ever-present flat hat in greeting, always referring to her as "Mrs. Billington," but when he entered our house or clinic, he immediately removed his hat. Like Peter, his friend Andrew Kunnizzi and the old chief Johnny Kay were all kind and polite men, thoughtful to everyone, and they were also humble, a personality trait that Mary Teya also carried, as did her father, John Tetlitchi, who had been the chief for many years.

Later that day Peter, Don and I had stopped at another camp where a tent had been set up, and Peter went in for a brief visit. However, Don and I were eager to move on before it got too late. It was after four-thirty in the afternoon when we knocked on the door of Brian Francis's cabin at Three Cabin Creek, close to the mouth of Vittrekwa Creek. The dogs were tired and didn't need to be tied up. They just curled up where they were in the snow, tucking their noses deep into their warm fur.

Brian Francis came out of his cabin, an ever-present cigarette in his mouth, to invite us inside and, as was customary, offered us moose meat, bannock and tea, which we readily accepted. But while it was Brian who offered us the supper, it was his wife who glided

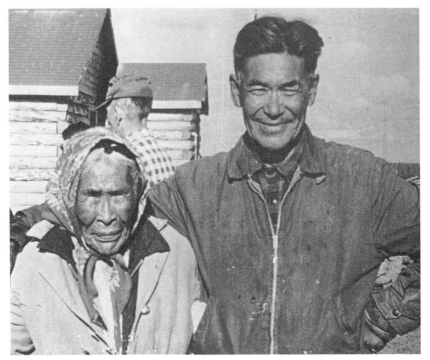

Brian Francis, a lively old man, stands with Old Harriet Stewart, a village elder. FRANK DUNN PHOTO.

silently around the cabin in her moccasins, moving from one wood stove to another as she prepared the refreshments for us. She was a big woman, and whenever any comments were made to her, she would just smile and nod in agreement and then move on to continue her work. The addition of a few split logs on the fire soon had it crackling with life, and the kettle, filled with pieces of ice from the river, started to spit and hiss as the ice melted.

Suddenly I noticed the form of someone lying on a bed in a dark corner of the cabin. "Who's that?" I asked, indicating the person who lay covered with a sleeping bag.

"Sarah. She got bad teeth and doesn't feel too good."

Their daughter Sarah had come to the clinic several times, complaining of a nagging toothache and pointing to her top front teeth. As she was only in her early twenties, I had refused to pull out the

offending teeth because I thought that pulling them would disfig-
ure her, and I cherished the hope that a dentist would soon visit
the village. Now she was feeling miserable as the pills that I had
given her in the clinic no longer alleviated her pain. I could smell
the oil of cloves that she had used in a vain attempt to assuage the
pain, and now when I went over to her, she asked me if I would
reconsider pulling out her teeth. As it was close to breakup, there
was no possibility that a dentist would be coming to the village for
another two months—even if then—and I could not let her suffer
for all that time.

It was still light outside, but inside the cabin with its low roof I
would not be able to see very much, especially in someone's mouth.
However, Brian lit a gas lamp for me and set it on the table, and
Sarah came to sit beside it. As usual I had a basic set of instruments with me, and after I had injected the local anaesthetic, ex-
tracting the teeth was easy for me and painless for Sarah. A few
minutes later she was showing her mother the gap in her smile.
She seemed to bounce back from her earlier misery very quickly,
but I gave her some strong pain pills to take when the anaesthetic
wore off. I always found that this sort of dentistry, although crude,
not only gave the patient satisfaction but me as well, because I was
able to make the patient's life more tolerable.

While we were in the cabin, the wind started blowing fiercely
down the river, and when we went outside, we discovered that the
blowing snow had almost made the far side of the river disappear.
Brian suggested that, as it was getting late, we should stay with them
overnight, and perhaps the weather would improve by morning. Peter was in no hurry to go anywhere in a raging storm, so after making sure that the dogs were well bedded down, we returned to the
cabin with our sleeping bags and found places for them on the cabin
floor. Above the sound of the stove crackling away, we could hear the
wind whistling around the eaves of the cabin, and the fact that we
were so well sheltered made me feel quite comfortable, even though
I was lying on the wooden planks of an uneven floor. There was some

conversation then silence as Brian tuned into radio station CHAK for "Neighbourly News and Messages." When it was finished, Brian turned off the radio, put out the gas lamp and with a "good night" echoing from each of us, we settled down to sleep. After a hard day on the trail in the biting cold, going to sleep early was easy in the comfort of a warm and dark cabin.

As often happens after a high wind, during the night the temperature had dropped right down to minus thirty-five (C). It was blowing from the north, so we were doomed to face it all the way home. After a breakfast of fried caribou meat and bannock, we waved farewell to Brian and his wife, and Sarah came to say that she had slept well for the first time in weeks.

Once we were down on the river, my dogs followed Peter's team, and periodically I jumped off my toboggan and ran for a short while to try to stay warm. It was hard to breathe deeply when jogging because the freezing cold air would freeze either my nostrils or, if I breathed through my mouth, my throat. And when I rode on the back of the toboggan, I tried to keep my head turned slightly to one side so that the wind did not blow directly into my parka hood where it seemed to penetrate my toque. I also fastened my scarf around my neck in an attempt to keep the fur-trimmed hood closer to my skin.

I thought of my peers who worked down south in warm hospitals, men and women walking around in their crisp white uniforms. Did I envy them? I asked myself. Would I like to trade their circumstances for mine, riding behind a dog team down a cold but beautiful river, clothed with Gwich'in-made mukluks and parka, listening to the bells on the dog harness tinkling as they plodded along? No, I realized. I was cold but I was free.

Weeks later the ice broke up and moved out, but one day before the river ran entirely free of ice a scow pulled up to the bank below the nursing station and Sarah Francis came up to the clinic. Without hesitation she came up to me and said quietly, "Dad died a few days ago up at the cabin but we couldn't get down because of the ice." This was a complete shock to me. Brian was an old man but he was lively, one of the men at Christmastime who had danced the most, and when we saw him up at the cabin before breakup he had seemed vigorous enough.

"What happened, Sarah?" I couldn't keep the surprise out of my voice. "He seemed fine when we saw him just a few weeks ago."

"I know," Sarah said softly. "He got a bad cough and it got worse and worse until he had a bad fever. I thought about trying to walk down, but it was too hard with the ice being so soft, and we didn't know when it was going to break up." She looked down at the floor, and I could imagine the anguish that she and her mother must have felt as they saw Brian getting worse. "We couldn't get him to drink and then after a couple of days he died."

"Well, Sarah," I told her, "I'll look after your dad now. I'll have to let the police know and they may want to talk to you, but don't worry—they only want the details that you just told me. I'll let Don Wootten know at the church and he'll be around to see you, too."

When the family had gone, we arranged for Brian's body to be carried on a stretcher to one of the outbuildings behind the nursing station that we referred to as "igloos" because of their shape. I went to prepare Brian for burial, washing and dressing him and combing his hair. Then while I waited for someone to bring the cloth-covered coffin to put him in, I found myself talking to the dead man. "Brian," I said, "why did you do this?" I knew it was silly to talk to a lifeless man but I wanted to break the silence. "Now what is your family going to do?" Who was going to get the meat for them? Who would do the trapping to earn cash? Of course, I knew that the Indian agent would make sure that Brian's wife and daughter were materially looked after, but I grieved for them, and for Brian, because the change in their way of life was going to be so very difficult.

CHAPTER FIVE

URIEL AND I WERE VERY FORTUNATE to have lived in Fort McPherson before many of the big changes occurred that were to alter the way of life of the Gwich'in people so irrevocably. But while at that time we considered their lives to be romantic and full of adventure, the reality for the people who lived that old way was a life fraught with danger, hardship and quite often hunger. Of course, we never thought of ourselves as instruments of change, but as we tried to teach public health principles, that is what we were actually endeavoring to do—change the habits, customs and some of the beliefs that had been handed down from generation to generation. The schoolteachers were also trying to instill the principles of the white man's world into young children, and all of us believed that what we were doing would improve the lot of the Gwich'in. Who could argue with better houses and sanitation? Education and health? A welfare system that would take care of the elderly and single families? These were all ideals, but they would change forever a traditional way of life where the chief made all the decisions for the band, where families were responsible for individual members, and where the elders taught the young people where and when the animals that they relied on for food could be found.

The Gwich'in people had been nomadic, following the great caribou herds in the mountains in wintertime and descending to the rivers that were abundant with fish in the summertime. Everything they used—moss diapers, skin clothing, fresh or dried meat, smoked fish—was disposable. Sanitation had not been a problem and campsites soon returned to their natural state. But how many Europeans would like to live as their ancestors had, cooking over smoky coal fires, emptying their "night pails" out of the window where the contents ran into a stinking sewer in the centre of the cobbled road? When transportation was by horse or on foot, and foods were generally so rancid that they had to be heavily spiced to disguise their taste?

The romantic picture disappears rapidly, and this was the conclusion that we had come to as we saw changes occurring, very slowly but still definite, among the Gwich'in, and we had to agree that in this modern day and age progress would continue and ultimately benefit all northern people. Yet, as one distinguished chief told us, "It is education that is spoiling the people. Now they don't go out on the land, they don't attend band meetings, and then they criticize the council for decisions that they make."

The new Chief Julius School had just opened its doors a few days before our arrival in Fort McPherson in 2009, but we did not have an opportunity to visit it. Back in the early sixties there had been just one school in the community, the Peter Warren Dease School, and it was operated by the Department of Northern Affairs. The children who were attending could live at home. They were expected to stay in Fleming Hall, the children's hostel in the village, when their parents went out to the camps for hunting and trapping, but as soon as their parents came back to the village, if only for the weekend, the children were supposed to go home. An annex had been built to accommodate the growing number of children, and plans were being made to build a newer, bigger school, but the start date for that was sometime in the next decade.

In those days the children could start in the beginners class and go through to grade 8, but to continue their schooling, they had to go to Inuvik. There the Fort McPherson contingent stayed at Stringer Hall, an Anglican-run hostel, while the children from Arctic Red River stayed at a Roman Catholic-run hostel. Young people who wanted to take vocational training had to go to Yellowknife, hundreds of kilometres to the south. This had all been carefully planned out by a benevolent government, but it caused conflict for the Gwich'in people who for centuries had survived as closely knit family units, relying on their young folk to help with the hunting, trapping, moving camp, gathering wood and all the other activities that made their survival in the bush possible.

Whenever I visited camps out in the Delta or up in the Richardson Mountains, there were only very young children present with the adults, and it seemed as though a whole generation was missing from that environment. And the parents resented having to send their children to the hostels in Inuvik for a high school education, especially when the children had to be away from September to June with only short visits home at Christmas and Easter. They said that they lost control of the youngsters too soon and that, when the children came home for the holidays, they wouldn't do anything to help around the home, and the adults feared that their old way of life, which had been carried on for centuries, would soon end.

In a column published in the Inuvik newspaper *The Drum* in July 1966, writer Wallace Labillois commented on the Indian Pavilion at Expo 67 and what kind of story it should tell the world. He said:

Many Indians [in Canada] feel that education can be an important key to the future—they feel, however, that Indian children are under a considerable handicap in relation to non-Indians. School curricula and text books are usually designed for children of a European background and have very little relationship to the Indian child's home experience—schools are organized according to a strict, European time schedule which is alien to Indian tradition. In some cases he learns to be ashamed of his own culture. In many cases, Indian children have to travel considerably greater distances to school than non-Indian children. Often they are removed from their home communities for considerable periods of time in residential schools which are an alien environment. They are often estranged from their family and their community when they return home …

The Indian is in a turmoil, he is grasping the future with one hand while with the other he is holding fast on to the values he wants to keep from his past. If he is going to adapt successfully to modern life, he will have to pull as hard with one hand as with the other.

This was all true in Fort McPherson where, after their formal education was completed, those youngsters who returned to the village had to reintegrate into the community where all the professional jobs, such as game warden, police, school teacher, nurse, electrician, the Indian agent and even Anglican minister and the Roman Catholic priest, were filled by white people from Outside. One of the causes of conflict, especially for the girls coming back to their home community, was their dress. Miniskirts had become popular in the south by this time, and fashion-conscious young Gwich'in women would come back from Yellowknife or Edmonton with short skirts, tight leather boots and loose tops, and everyone found that it was hard to look them in the eye! Before long even the boys wanted to wear thin zippered coats and no hat even in winter. Traditional clothing was completely ignored if not forgotten. Fortunately the children who stayed in Fleming Hall were brought to the hostel in appropriate clothing or the hostel staff provided them with adequate clothing.

The Gwich'in traditionally used caribou skins for their attire and dressed their children in caribou calfskins, which are soft and pliable. Mukluks made from caribou leg skin were ideal for springtime use because, with the hair left on the hide, they shed the wet snow just as that skin had shed it for the original owners. However, the returning young people preferred white man's clothing now, and as the weather cooled off rapidly in the fall, there was a sharp contrast between what they were wearing and what we transient white people wore. We had adapted happily to long underwear, heavy pants

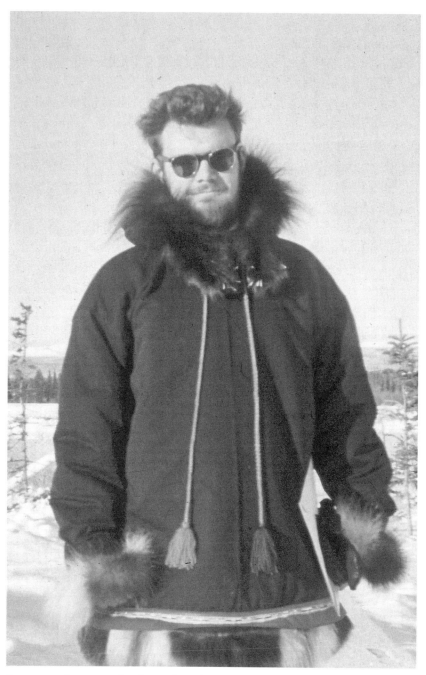

I was proud to wear fur-fringed parkas and hide mukluks.

and thick shirts and were proud to wear fur-fringed parkas and hide mukluks. Even in the summertime we covered ourselves up for protection from the hordes of mosquitoes and blackflies who were determined to suck our blood dry.

One year, a visiting dentist, Dr. Bob Ruzika—who was known as the Mackenzie Singing Dentist or the Mackenzie Bard—stayed with us in the nursing station for several weeks and confided to Muriel that he really wanted a pair of pants made from caribou hide. Muriel offered to make him a pair if the right kind and quantity of hide could be obtained, and by coincidence Bob discovered that the Indian agent stocked some very soft deer hide for sale to Gwich'in women who used it in their handicrafts. With lots of patience and after several broken sewing machine needles, Muriel completed the pants for a very satisfied customer, and during Bob's stay we enjoyed his guitar-playing and singing in the evenings.

When a group of nine Gwich'in men, a Metis man and myself were preparing to make a dog team trip to Dawson City in the Yukon, the older women in the village made each of us caribou skin parkas. They used the caribou summer skins, cutting them in such a way that the finished product had a handsome design and hand sewing them together with sinew. I found mine to be extremely warm even at forty below.

When we came back in 2009, we noticed that there were now satellite dishes on most of the roofs and big television sets in the houses, and we wondered if television was having a detrimental effect on the culture and way of life of the people. We visited Abe Stewart in his home and he told us he was now an elder and had been interviewed by a group who were trying to assess some of the changes in the Gwich'in lifestyle. He gave us a copy of the interview transcript in which he said that "people don't go anywhere if they have to walk!" There is no doubt that, although the diet of the Tetlit Gwich'in has improved in quality and no one starves to death anymore, a common phenomenon a hundred or more years ago, the increased quantity of food in conjunction with a lack of exercise is causing some major problems with over-weight people and an alarming increase in diabetic cases.

The Gwich'in had not used dog teams until white people intro-duced them into the country when they were pushing north to the goldfields at the end of the nineteenth century, no doubt to the relief of the Gwich'in women, who had previously done all the work as-sociated with moving camp. In the early sixties most of the people still travelled by dog team, and I never quite lost my excitement and wonderment when I saw a team of dogs go past our living room window with the bells on the harnesses jingling and the driver bal-ancing on the toboggan, the back of his parka encrusted with glis-tening snow crystals. Finally, six months after our arrival in Fort McPherson, having now decided that we would stay indefinitely, I made up my mind to get a dog team of my own. Up to this time I had been using dog teams made up mostly of a few spare dogs from a person here and a person there, a combination that was sure to cause some conflict. I bought three pups from Lucy Rat early in the spring of 1964 and was given two pups by the RCMP. (Later on I obtained two more from them.) I kept them penned up on the grounds of the nursing station behind our outbuildings so that they would not be too obvious to any visiting officials. By the follow-ing fall I tried putting them into harness and that turned out to be a trial of patience and perseverance. But once out on the trail, the pups—because that is what they were really with their long legs and slim bodies, more like gangly teenagers—seemed to call up their sled dog genes and actually ran in some sort of formation down the river trail. Then as soon as the trail had been made to the Mouth of the Peel, I took them for a run down to the cabins there. They arrived exhausted, but that was a good thing because they did not have the energy to romp around. By the time I got them home again, I felt that I had the makings of a good team.

❄ ❄ ❄

There were already a few snowmobiles in the village by that time, though they would be hard to associate with the sleek and powerful

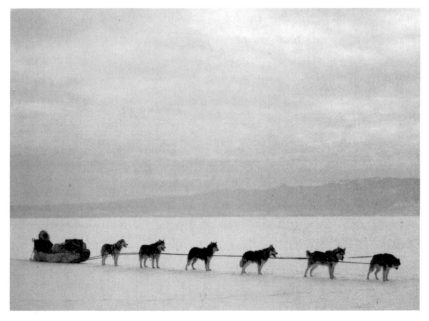

Muriel is all packed up and rarin' to go in a loaded toboggan!

models that became popular by the end of the century. And who could blame the men who instead of travelling for two or three days by dogsled to the caribou camps could make the same journey by snowmobile and bring back a load of meat in just two days? There were also a few trucks of various sizes and three Caterpillar tractors, the largest, the size of a D8, being renowned for digging itself into the melting permafrost to the top of its tracks. The old moosehide skin boats were long gone, mostly because the Gwich'in did not spend their winters in the upper reaches of the Peel River or in the Richardson and Ogilvie mountains anymore. Now outboard motors had become common, and some of the old Gwich'in men managed to putter along using a Seagull three-and-a-half horsepower motor—or "kicker"—on the back end of their long, flat-bottomed boats, loaded with wife, children, dogs, tents and camp supplies. Others, usually those in the younger set, were progressing by that time to twenty and thirty-five horsepower motors and some even larger.

Still, there was always something new for us to learn, gradually giving us a broader perspective on the northern way of life. Things that we had taken for granted when we lived Outside were nowhere to be found and we had to adapt to our new environment. I remember a teacher at the village's only school telling me that he was using educational material from the south, and one of the questions asked of his elementary pupils was "Where do you get your mail?" Of course, the answer in southern communities is the post office, but in nearly all the northern settlements the answer would be the Hudson's Bay store!

For Muriel and me, window shopping and browsing through the stores on a Friday evening changed to catalogue shopping, grocery shopping was done annually, and banking was done either by mail or through the Bay. Cash, however, hardly ever crossed our palms. When we went to any of the stores or to the Bay to make a purchase, we charged it to our account, and then at the end of the month, if we remembered or were reminded by the store manager, we paid with a cheque. When we rented equipment for personal use, such as a dog team or snowmobile, we often paid with groceries or traded for something that was of value to the renter. Any paper money that was used circulated around and around in the village until the notes became so crinkled and dirty that they were frequently referred to as "Dirty Delta Dollars."

Credit was synonymous with "owe." To decide how much credit to extend, the Bay manager would assess each person according to his wages, monthly social welfare income, Old Age Pension, past history of trapping good quality fur and record of paying his accounts. In the old days the unit of value was not the dollar but the "made beaver," based on the value of a prime beaver skin in excellent condition, and store goods were then priced at this rate. This brought the company's accounting practices into line with the Native bartering system and allowed the Bay's traders to issue a "grubstake" of the necessary food and supplies to people who were going out into the bush for seasonal trapping. When they returned, the value of the furs they delivered to the company was deducted from the amount owing and then more supplies given accordingly. Those trappers who had done well and still had credit available were referred to as being able to "get ahead."

It was the gold seekers who came through the Peel River country on their way to the Yukon goldfields who introduced money to the Gwich'in. Richard Slobodin, in his *Polar Notes*, tells of a popular Peel River tale called "How the People Learned about Money":

> *It is related that in the summer of 1899 a group of Peel River men, led by Chief Francis, tracked up the Rat River the boats of a party of gold seekers under the leadership of a certain Mr. Miller "from Chicago." To the Gwich'in of that period, Chicago seems to have been synonymous with the United States and a good deal of southern Canada. When they reached Mac-Dougall Pass, the stampeders attempted to pay the Indians off in cash instead of the agreed-upon trade goods. The Gwich'in demurred. Mr. Miller then paid them off with clothing, ammunition and other items. In addition, he presented each of the natives with some samples of currency.*
>
> *Most of this money was scattered sportively along the trail across the hills back to Fort McPherson. Some tore theirs up; others preserved a few bills as curiosities. One day a trader, corroborating the stampeders' claims, offered them goods for the paper stuff. The story goes that the young Indians staged a minor "rush" of their own, retracing their steps to search the muskeg for bits and pieces of the discarded bills.[1]*

One old man told me, "Indians don't have a bank, but the people—the Peel River people—is like a bank for us. You work all your life and help other people, and when you get old, everybody helps you." Maybe there was some wishful thinking in this remark, but maybe it was also a reminder to the young people that they had an obligation to the old people. Some of the older Gwich'in men, mainly those who had spent most of their time in the bush away from the village, did not really understand where white people obtained their money. One of them told me that if I wanted to buy something—in this case I was hiring a helicopter—all I had to do was "sign cheque." Bank accounts meant nothing to him, neither did the fact that we had jobs that we were paid to do. From his point of view he also worked—though at fishing and trapping and hunting—but he didn't get a government cheque. (He did later when he became eligible for the old-age pension.)

The world outside was still a strange place to the older Gwich'in, and world affairs meant very little to people who were involved with the hard work of surviving. During a social meeting I had with some white people and Gwich'in elders, we discussed some of the problems that arose between white people and Natives because neither fully understood the other side. One elder stated that white people had it really easy—they came North, had good houses and best of all they had "government cheque"—but the recipients of these cheques sometimes looked down on the poor Indians who had nothing. Another elder asked if people were like that where Muriel and I came from. "Who do they look down on over there?"

"Over in England we're all the same," I said.

"No," the man insisted, "who are the *Indians* in England?"

It was a difficult question to answer because we knew that there was class distinction among the whites in Britain and there was also prejudice by some against people of colour. However, as we became familiar with different families in Fort McPherson, it struck us that there were possibly social classes among the Gwich'in. It was apparent that some individuals from certain families would not, or could not, marry into other families. Some individuals had more intellectual discernment than others and took care of themselves and what they had, perhaps better than some others who lived in squalor and neglected their families. Anthropologists writing about Peel River people said that:

Mutual joking can take place between an adult and his or her brothers-in-law, sisters-in-law, cousins and grandparents. At all times an effort is made to assert as close a relationship as possible with persons of relatively high status. As the maintenance of high status requires the support of kin, this tendency is generally reciprocated. This means that, in effect, high ranking "wealthy" persons have many kin while poverty [means a] lack of kin.

Of course, we were not told of some of the social niceties among the Gwich'in and we had to learn them from observation. I learned that it was not proper for a man to tease a woman at all as that could be seen as having "an interest" in her. Now and again William Firth, who was a font of knowledge, would hint at certain aspects of social correctness and I don't think that he was breaking a Gwich'in confidence. Of course, he was officially "non-Native" because, although his mother was Gwich'in, his father was a Scot.

There were several instances when I became aware of the superstitious beliefs of the Gwich'in. Once when I was out fishing with a young man from Fort McPherson and we had gone downriver in his scow, he brought out his new shotgun to show me. I had never fired a shotgun so he loaded it and told me to fire away. Just then a raven flew over squawking noisily, and thinking that one less raven would be a good thing, I aimed the shotgun at it but before I could pull the trigger I was pushed and told in a loud voice, "Don't shoot! If you shoot a raven, we'll have really bad weather and we won't make it home!" He was convinced that ravens had the reincarnated spirit of a bad person who could change the weather so that we would have a catastrophe on the way home. And of course, ravens could make some strange sounds, like a stone rattling down an empty pipe or a gurgling squawk or an irritated caw, noises that sometimes sounded half-human. Another supposed cause of bad weather was a death in the community, so shortly after someone had died, we were told that we could expect the weather to deteriorate. It usually did anyway, whether anyone had died or not.

Some of the Gwich'in superstitions were not unique to them. Many cultures believe in a bogeyman or some other evil character that will come out and get you at an unexpected moment, and many a child has been told that he will be caught by one if he strays from home. It was old Harriet Stewart who first told us about the Gwich'in equivalent. When she turned up at the clinic one day in our first winter in Fort McPherson, we told her to come into the treatment room, but her weathered face broke into a smile and she pointed toward the kitchen with her walking stick, which was as brown and wrinkled as she was. "No sick, I come to visit. Tea!" she said emphatically and without any hesitation she set off down the corridor toward the kitchen.

We looked at each other, smiled, and Muriel said, "Why not? There's no one else waiting so let's join her!"

It was always a pleasure to have a visit from one of the elders, although it was sometimes difficult to follow their conversation because it was in broken English, but we could usually get the gist of their stories. Maria Snowshoe was our housemaid in the nursing station at that time, and she put both the teakettle and the coffee pot on when she saw us heading her way. Maria told Harriet in Gwich'in to sit down and said that tea would soon be ready. Harriet made herself comfortable, then looking at Maria, she nodded and said, "Aha, aha." Like all the older Gwich'in women who visited, she took off neither her parka nor her headscarf while inside the house.

"You go out in the bush?" she asked us, her head bobbing slightly, showing that her Parkinsonism was not controlled. She was letting us know that the village moccasin telegraph had circulated the news that these young nurses liked to get out and about.

"Yes, we walked down the trail past the dock and we want to visit some other places, too."

"You be careful. You never know what's in the bush."

I assumed she meant bears or wolves or some other predator.

"You know Nana-ee?" Harriet asked then, and I saw Maria smile and hide her mouth behind her hand.

"No, what is it?" I asked, sipping the coffee that Maria handed me.

"Bushman!" she said smilingly "But don't laugh. Lots of people see Bushman!"

"Is he from around here?"

"No, he is not Indian. He's big and wears sort of white man clothes. Big hat, too. Lives in Bush all time. We call him Nana-ee."

"We'll be careful, Harriet," Muriel said with a smile. "Thank you for telling us."

Harriet sat drinking her tea in silence and then got up to go. "Thanks for tea. That Maria, she take good care of you."

After she had gone, we asked Maria if Harriet had come just to tell us about the bushman.

"I guess so," she said. "Those old people really believe it."

"Do you?" Muriel asked.

"I dunno. That's what they say."

When William Firth came in, I asked him about the bushman. I couldn't tell if he believed in these things himself as he often referred to what "they"—the Native people—believed when he repeated the local legends. Now he told us, "He is about eight feet tall and wears a dress suit, you know, like they wear at fancy dinners. And he has a top hat, too."

Immediately my mind jumped to the old photos I had seen of the early explorers who had dressed up whenever they visited a Native camp, and I knew that the chief factors of the Hudson's Bay Company had dressed up formally whenever the superintendent and his retinue arrived at the post because they all wanted to impress each other as well as the Natives. These white men were invariably taller and heavier than the local Gwich'in men, and because of their power and prestige in the community they may have seemed larger than life. I could well imagine Gwich'in parents telling their children that one of these men would take them away if they didn't behave. Later, when I was travelling alone in the bush in the dark or when my dog team was the last in a line of teams, I had the feeling that someone or something was following me and

I could feel the hairs on my neck bristling. I was more concerned with wolves than with a bushman, but now and again I did glance behind me just for reassurance.

In a paper titled "Some Social Functions of Kutchin [Gwich'in] Anxiety," published in *The American Anthropologist* in February 1960, anthropologist Richard Slobodin explained that the Gwich'in belief in a bushman was a local form of a superstition that was widely spread among northern Athapascan tribes. This seemed to be confirmed by the fact that while some people told us that the bushman was tall, others thought he was a dwarf. Some also said he was half-human and half-supernatural and, though not very powerful, still to be considered a menace.

Apparently, the basis for a belief in a bushman was embedded into Gwich'in culture, because in the past if a lone person survived a tragedy, he would separate himself from the community and live on the fringes of society. It was the opinion of James Simon, a well-respected Gwich'in elder and church catechist, that in cases where a partnership was severed by an accidental death or starvation, "It's bad to be the one left alive. That's what we think." And it is true that expressions of anxiety for the lone survivor or an isolated small group of survivors are common in Peel River folklore.

Many Gwich'in stories tell of physical hardships or death through privation, and Slobodin was even told that "a story is no good without starvation in it." And there seems to have been a tendency for people in the old days to draw together in the face of death as a tightly knit group or remain together to await their end, and it is suggested that several place names in the Peel River area came about because a number of families starved and died together in those locations. However, if a few people or a single individual from that group survived, they would separate themselves from the rest of the community as though they were to be held accountable for the deaths of the others.

We were told that many years earlier in the Mackenzie Delta a motorboat was destroyed by a gasoline explosion, killing the four young men riding in it. Two bodies were found and identified quite quickly and a third was found some weeks later, damaged beyond identification. When it was announced that this third body had been found, the relatives of both missing men claimed it without having seen it, and both families turned out in force for the inquest. Because of their conflicting testimony, the coroner's jury found that there was not enough evidence and failed to declare an identification.

As time went on and the fourth body was not found, rumours began to circulate that one or the other of the missing men had been seen, implying that the unidentified body must be that of the other family's son. No one would accept the conclusion of the RCMP that there had been no survivors, but after a few months one of the families seemed to have gained the popular vote that the third body was that of their son, and the opposing family gave up. Meanwhile, the young man who was believed to have survived was rumored to have been seen further and further south. Even ten years later two men from the Peel River said that they had seen him at the Calgary Stampede, but when approached he had disappeared. Such was the stigma for any survivor.

In another incident a man from another village offered to take a fourteen-year-old Gwich'in boy to hunt muskrat in the Mackenzie Delta where there is a myriad of lakes and portages. They became separated, and when the older man was unable to find the boy, he made his way to the main river channel where he found a Gwich'in chief and implored him and his party to help search for the boy. The members of this camp were in the middle of hunting muskrat themselves, but eventually the chief sent out a search party, and after two days of combing the lakesides, portages and trails, they spotted the youth in the thick bush. However, as it was known that some people, after being lost in the bush, would sometimes run off and become lost again when approached by a group of searchers, when this lad was sighted, everyone stopped and waited until the chief could approach him alone and quietly. Later the older hunter admitted that he had never felt so good in all his life as when they found the boy. He had been scared that if the boy had not been found, he would have been under suspicion of foul play, especially as he was from another village. But in spite of all the rumour and gossip surrounding survivors, the Gwich'in were said to be against openly expressing hostility to them.

CHAPTER SIX

L IVING AND WORKING IN A REMOTE village, looking after the health—or more precisely the illnesses—of the Gwich'in people, had the tendency to make Muriel and me appear hard and unemotional, or at least that is what we assumed must be the case. Neither of us attended funerals, and when tragedy struck or an emergency occurred, we worked hard to maintain a calm exterior so that we could respond appropriately and function properly. But holding in our personal emotions was sometimes quite a strain, and many times my throat would literally ache when, for instance, a baby or young child died and we could see and feel the grief of the parents and experience our own sense of inadequacy.

One little girl who was obviously very ill was brought to the nursing station. Her breathing was shallow, she was quite pale and her skin was cold and clammy. According to her mother, she had not been well all day, and then when she went to check on her, "She looked just like that." There were many questions that I would have liked to have asked about what was happening in the house during the day and how closely the little girl was watched, but these things were not important at that moment. Muriel and I X-rayed the child's chest then applied warm blankets and an oxygen mask before inserting an IV and monitoring her temperature, but she lay quietly, eyes closed, barely breathing. Together we hung over her, watching.

"She's stopped breathing!" Muriel almost shouted and immediately started to try to resuscitate her. I used a positive pressure bag attached to an oxygen cylinder to force some oxygen into her lungs. Desperately we continued until we could see that the little life had gone, but even then it was some time before we looked at each other and silently gave up.

"Why?" The question was asked of no one in particular. "What could we have done that we didn't do?" We felt angry and upset at our inability to help. The child's death had been so sudden and without any apparent reason. When we calmed down, we sent for William, and after telling him what had happened, sent him with a message for the parents to come down to the clinic. William just nodded and left the station quietly.

I knew that I would have to break the news of their daughter's death to them and try to explain something that I didn't even know the answer to myself. Together Muriel and I would comfort them as well as we could, and they would inevitably cry as would the other family members, while Muriel and I would hold our own grief in until everyone had gone. Then we would have to keep a cool composure as the little girl was carried out and sent to Inuvik by plane because an autopsy would have to be done to find out the cause of death, and all the time we would be feeling guilty because we hadn't saved her life. Later we would have to remind each other that we were there to help where help was possible, but we could not control life.

One evening a baby girl was brought into the clinic by a distraught mom who said that her daughter had been fussy all day, crying nonstop, and nothing seemed to satisfy her. She had given the child some infant fever medicine even though the little girl did not seem to be feverish, bathed her and settled her for the night, but a very short time later she woke up again crying.

Both Muriel and I examined the little patient. She had a very slight fever but no other signs of illness. As Muriel surveyed our drug cupboard's contents, she said, "She must be cooking something," meaning that she was probably incubating some bacteria or a virus.

We did not like to prescribe antibiotics when there was no significant diagnosis, but we decided that a broad spectrum antibiotic might clear up any potential chest infection, and we gave the mother a bottle of children's antibiotic medicine. We told her to continue with the fever medicine as well and said we would see her the following day. Early the next morning when we opened the clinic waiting room door, the same mom came in with her daughter.

"She didn't sleep hardly at all last night, just cried and cried," she said, "and she won't take her bottle either and she just spits out the medicine that you gave me for her."

We could see that the mother was tired and worried. Muriel and I conferred and decided to admit the baby to the nursing station where we could watch and treat her. The mother was relieved when we told her this. "Come back and see her anytime but first go home and rest." Muriel put her hand on the young mom's arm and led her to the door.

We put the baby into a crib and examined her again. She was moderately dehydrated and quite irritable, but she had no chest sounds or cough, no diarrhea, no tender abdomen, nothing to give us a clue about her condition. We decided that first of all we must get some fluid into her, but when Muriel tried feeding her apple juice, then water, all the child did was turn her head from side to side and cry.

When we called the hospital, the doctor confirmed that it was very important to get some liquid into the little patient. He suggested either a scalp intravenous or, if that didn't work, we could use a syringe and put some water into the child's rectum or inject some sterile water interstitially, that is, under the skin. "As soon as the weather improves in Inuvik, we'll send a plane. Let us know how you get on." Then he hung up.

There are special fine needles for giving scalp infusions, and with Muriel holding the baby's arms, I successfully got the needle into a tiny vein and taped the plastic tubing to her forehead.

Muriel then gave her an injection of a pediatric antibiotic and held the little girl on her knee, trying to comfort her so that she would not try to reach up to the IV.

Fortunately, the weather improved in late afternoon and we sent the baby to the Inuvik General Hospital with the nurse who flew in to escort her. The mother said that she had to stay in the village to look after the rest of her young family.

When patients were sent to Inuvik or Edmonton for medical reasons, there were always numerous forms to be made out by hand and sent along with them. Children who were sent out often went unescorted by their parents, although they were in the care of an adult while they were on the plane and were met by hospital staff in Inuvik. Attached to them were stiff brown envelopes containing all of their personal information, just as though they were human parcels.

The forms that we had to complete must have had their origin in some southern hospital and been merely adapted for northern communities in order to obtain information on their Indian status. Ever since Treaty #11 had been signed in June 1921, each individual Gwich'in person had a band number, a family number and a personal number, and then in the early sixties when Social Insurance Numbers (SIN) were introduced, they acquired one more number. For the Gwich'in, having an actual name must have seemed superfluous! However, we often laughed as we filled in the questions asking for distinguishing features such as colour of hair and eyes. Of the Gwich'in people in Fort McPherson, 99 percent had black hair, brown eyes and a dark complexion. In fact, whenever we saw a group of the young children from the hostel all together, they were as alike as peas in a pod—same haircut, same clothes, same sparkling smiles!

But as we got to know individual children and adults, we began to distinguish the facial characteristics of the different Gwich'in families, although we had to be careful not to comment on this because there was always the possibility of upsetting someone if the father was "unknown." On the other hand, there never seemed to be "unwanted" children in Fort McPherson, and at an earlier time babies from one family were sometimes given to another family to raise, or a young child would be given to grandparents so that there would be someone to care for them in their old age. In this way the Gwich'in had their own Children and Family Services long before the bureaucracy became involved.

Our little patient had been admitted to the children's ward at the Inuvik hospital, and later when we inquired about her, we were told that no diagnosis had been made but that she remained in the same irritable condition. Four days later we had a call from Dr. Dave Wilkinson, the pediatrician we had known when we were working in the Charles Camsell Indian and Eskimo Hospital, who was visiting the Inuvik General Hospital in a consulting capacity.

"That little girl you sent in," he began, "I saw her and asked the doctor what her diagnosis was and he said that there wasn't one yet. They were waiting for blood test results, so I looked the little girl over, checked the chart and then told him right off that she had meningitis!" He went on to say that he had seen several young children down south with the same sort of atypical symptoms, so he had done a spinal tap on our little patient and his diagnosis was confirmed.

I asked why the antibiotic we had given her had not helped, and he explained that small doses would mask the symptoms but not treat the underlying cause. He had put her on massive doses of a special antibiotic and she was already improving. We were relieved that the patient was going to recover and hurried to pass the information on to the worried mother, but we felt badly that we had not recognized the disease at first and then had masked it by giving an antibiotic that was not appropriate. If we had ever felt proud of our abilities, it was this sort of thing that knocked the stuffing out of us. And it made us doubly careful when examining the little tykes who could not tell us exactly how they were feeling but only show by their behaviour that they were feeling ill.

❄ ❄ ❄

During a regular visit to Arctic Red River, Muriel examined a young woman named Martha whose term was getting close and advised her that she should get the next plane to Inuvik as this was where the women in that settlement were supposed to go for their confinement. But the patient was reluctant to go because she had other youngsters to care for, and Muriel surmised that she did not really trust her husband to care for them adequately. She sounded determined to stay in Arctic Red River to have her baby even though there was no one there to help her, but after much discussion Muriel persuaded her to come instead to Fort McPherson for the delivery because if all went well she could be home again in a few days. Martha brought her children with her and stayed with some friends in Fort McPherson until she went into labour and came down to the station. The delivery went off without a hitch and for the next few days she sat in bed doing some exquisite beadwork on a piece of moose skin and getting some rest from her daily chores at home.

While Muriel was busy with Martha, I did a clinic to which old Lucy Rat came complaining that ever since she had fallen into her woodpile she had great difficulty breathing. I examined her, took an X-ray of her chest and saw that she had broken some ribs. She lived alone and there was no one to care for her so I admitted her to the nursing station where she could be monitored and get some rest. "Tell Walter he better feed my dogs and those pups," she said as I helped her into bed.

Even with two patients to care for, we also had to continue our clinics, home visits and school health programs, and we were heading off for bed after a busy day when the doorbell rang just after midnight. Fortunately we had just discharged Martha, who was going to fly back to Arctic Red River the following day, because our midnight caller was another woman about to give birth. Beatrice Jerome was well into labour and we admitted her to the bed that Muriel and I had just remade after Martha's discharge. The new baby was born at

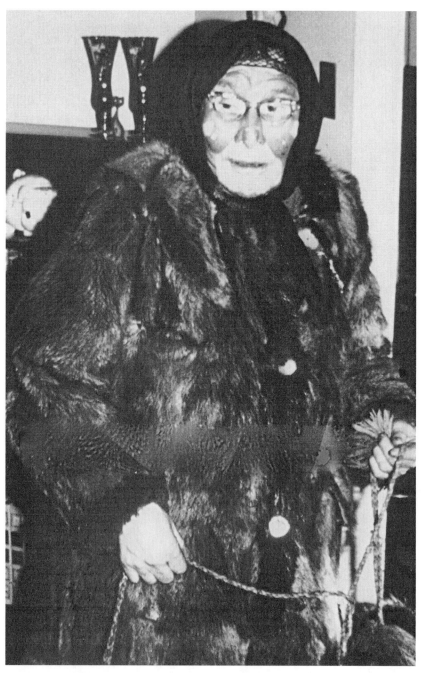

Old Lucy Rat was admitted to the nursing station with broken ribs.
FRANK DUNN PHOTO.

two in the morning, and it was after three by the time we were able to climb into bed, exhausted, but it was difficult to fall asleep because our senses were now tuned to the cry of the baby.

The next morning was a bright sunny day, and as Lucy was recovering, I took her for a short walk. I think that she enjoyed walking up to the village hanging onto my arm, and although she was mostly blind with cataracts and did not recognize people until they spoke, she was happy to return the greetings of those who hailed her. Later in the afternoon when Lucy was back in bed, Muriel went in to see her and asked if perhaps she could read to her. Lucy handed her a Bible and asked her to read some of that, but when Muriel opened it up, she discovered that it was in the Tukudh language of the Gwich'in! She did manage to read some of it though "very stumblingly," and Lucy responded by just nodding as Muriel read, and then in typical Gwich'in fashion she said, "Aha, aha" when the reading came to an end.

❄ ❄ ❄

Both Beatrice and Lucy were discharged a few days later, and then with the help of Rachel Stuart, the linens were washed, the rooms cleaned and the beds made. One of the beds was immediately needed for old Mary Neyendo who had to stay over with us for three consecutive nights to enable us to do some special tuberculosis tests on her. These had to be done first thing in the morning so there was no lying in bed to catch up on our sleep! When the last test was completed three days later we discharged her then stretched, yawned and had our breakfast, ready to face another day.

Eating a meal after doing some of the procedures that we had to do would seem very difficult but it rarely bothered us. During meals we would often discuss various diseases in detail and not think anything about it. Later when our children were old enough to listen in on our conversations, they took it all in stride, and it was something of a surprise to us to find that other people who joined us for meals were not particularly thrilled when the subject was gross anatomy.

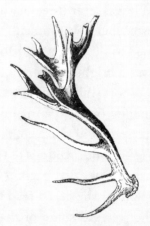

ROBERT MCDONALD WAS ONE OF THE important instruments of change on the Peel River. His father had come to Canada from Scotland to work for the "Honourable Company of Gentlemen Trading out of Hudson's Bay," but young Robert, born in 1829 on the Red River, was not destined to be a Bay man and chose the Anglican ministry instead. In 1862 he was assigned to the Yukon and then went further north as he tried to contact the nomadic Native people. At first he would converse with them through an interpreter but over the years he learned to speak the Tukudh language of the Gwich'in people. As their language had never been written down and McDonald's goal was to have the Bible available to them in their own language, he translated it and the Book of Common Prayer into Tukudh before preparing a grammar of the language as well. By 1873 McDonald, now the Anglican archbishop of the Mackenzie Diocese, was living in Fort McPherson where he taught basic English to both children and adults. When John Firth came to Fort McPherson in 1893 to look after the Bay's interests, he sometimes assisted McDonald in teaching English—which would have been interesting as his own tongue was Scots and he reputedly had a very broad accent!

CHAPTER SEVEN

C AROL McCORMACK, THE NURSE IN CHARGE of the William Firth Health Centre in 2009, said that her staff had
most of the equipment and supplies that were needed to
provide good treatment and a public health program. But when we
asked after some of the elders we had known, we were quite shocked
to learn that many of them, as well as many young people, had suc-
cumbed to cancer. For the size of the population there seemed to be
an inordinate number of cases, and yet we had never read or heard
any official outcry about this.

Carol said that they were also treating an increasing number of
diabetes cases, something that had not been prevalent amongst the
Gwich'in in the sixties when the biggest scourge among First Nations people throughout the North was tuberculosis. The Canadian
government had made some attempt to alleviate that problem by
doing X-ray surveys, tuberculin testing and vaccination, and whenever it was thought appropriate, hospitalizing positive or suspicious
cases. However, hospitalizing such patients was a double-edged
sword. As there were no tuberculosis hospitals in the North, patients
were sent to the Charles Camsell Hospital in Edmonton, or to the
Coqualeetza Hospital in Chilliwack, British Columbia. They were
thousands of kilometres from family, language and an environment
that they understood, and they had to remain there for many, many
years until their disease was controlled.

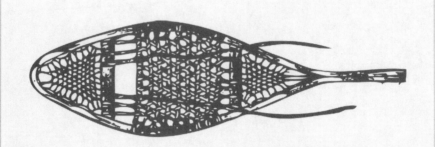

ON JUNE 27, 1921, THE FEDERAL government had signed treaties of a sort with the "northern Indians," a term which included the First Nations of Slave, Dogrib, Loucheux (Gwich'in), Hare and other people of the Northwest Territories north of Great Slave Lake. Under the terms of Treaty #11 these First Nations ceded a total of about 595,000 square kilometres of land to the government in exchange for "treaty presents" of "medals and flags" and a copy of the treaty for each chief, plus fishing, hunting and trapping equipment to the value of $50 for each family, as well as "miscellaneous equipment." There were also annual payments to band members: "Indians $5.00, chiefs $25.00, headmen $15.00; triennial suit of clothes to chiefs and headmen; annual distribution of twine, ammunition, etc." But the government wasn't really giving anything away because under the section of the treaty called "Government Obligations" it was stated that they would give "reserves one square mile for each family of five, subject to the government's right to deal with settlers on reserve lands; the right to sell or lease reserve lands with consent of Indians and to appropriate reserve lands for federal public purposes subject to compensation for improvements and lands; the right to hunt, trap and fish in ceded area subject to government regulations." In addition, the government agreed to "pay salaries of teachers."

The adults sometimes did handicrafts, but their minds were on their families back home in the North where men and women relied on each other for survival. Some of these older people never returned to the North. The children sent to these hospitals were first awed and then frightened. Most had never even heard of elevators and certainly had never been in one, so you can imagine the reaction of the northern child who was taken into a small room where the door closes, there's lots of noise and the little room shakes for a short time and then the door opens again but outside everything looks different. And when you have grown up with flush toilets and showers, it is at first amusing to see a northern child on his hands and knees in the bathroom looking to see where the contents of the toilet bowl went after he was shown how to flush. I was surprised one day to see a small boy cowering in the corner of a shower stall, staring at the small nozzle in the wall where water was spraying out and over him. He saw this as punishment, not a luxury!

Children in the Charles Camsell Hospital attended school there, and being young, soon picked up the English language, the common denominator among the many different languages spoken there. Then after years spent in these sterile surroundings and now only speaking English, they came to the end of their treatment and were sent home. The parents, who had sent out scrawny, sick five-year-olds, hardly recognized the well-fed, tall youths who emerged from the plane. And the returning child usually found himself in a crowded home, maybe sharing a bed with three or four more siblings, eating unfamiliar food and surrounded by people that he could not understand. It was not too surprising to us that some families would take off into the bush with their sick family member so he would not be whisked off to the south, possibly never to be seen again.

❄ ❄ ❄

To detect tuberculosis early, an X-ray survey team was sent out annually to all the settlements in the North, and in order to make sure that everyone was X-rayed, an arrangement was made for the team to travel with the annual "Treaty Party." This was a team of government

officials—including red-coated RCMP officers to keep law and order—that went to each village and with much pomp and ceremony
made payments to the Native people in accordance with the terms of
Treaty #11. After serious outbreaks of tuberculosis began to occur,
it was decided that treaty payments would not be made until each
person could show that he or she had been X-rayed. Fortunately,
by the time we arrived in the sixties this procedure had been abandoned, and the federal health services was sending an independent,
well-equipped X-ray team throughout the Northwest Territories
quite separate from the Treaty Party. And as the nursing stations
in most of the villages were now equipped with X-ray machines,
the doctors did not have to wait for a whole year when requesting
repeat chest X-rays.

Our aim was to schedule the survey in Fort McPherson for the
fall just before freeze-up when school was in full swing and most
of the Gwich'in people would still be in the village before going
out to their traplines. We put up posters in strategic places, and the
Anglican minister would even announce the dates and times at the
conclusion of his service. Of course, the teachers had to be advised
when the team would be arriving because the school routine would
be upset for several days. However, the team was at the mercy of the
weather, and if they couldn't get into one settlement, they would fly
into whichever area had the best weather.

One year, with freeze-up imminent, we were all set for the big
day, when we received a message that the survey team had been delayed. They would not be arriving that day but would come the following morning. The next day dawned clear and we geared up, ready
for a busy day, when another message came that they had been delayed again. All we could do was shrug and accept what was to be,
but we felt sorry for the schoolteachers who were trying to stick to
the curriculum. Then we received yet another message to say that,
as the team would be unable to get in the following day either, they
had cancelled the survey until after freeze-up. At this point we were
almost relieved and we let everyone know what was happening.

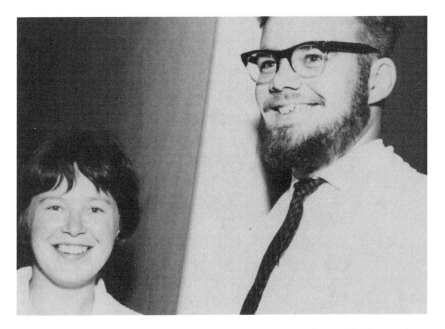

Muriel and I during a radiograph orientation at Camsell Hospital in Edmonton.

Imagine our surprise—and we weren't the only ones—when a messenger arrived from the school to tell us that the X-ray survey team had arrived after all and were already set up in the school and that there was a doctor with them, too! We dashed up to the school to invite the doctor to come to the nursing station as there were a few patients that we would like his advice on. He seemed rather surprised that he should be expected to see patients, and in the end we were quite happy when he returned to the school to watch the X-ray team at work.

Having most of the residents X-rayed was a good preventive program and could help to provide an early diagnosis, but it did mean that we were kept busy doing TB tests, vaccinations and repeat X-rays. Before going North, Muriel and I had spent almost a year working at the Charles Camsell Hospital in Edmonton, and after we had been identified as the future staff for Fort McPherson, we were given a brief but thorough orientation on procedures that nurses in

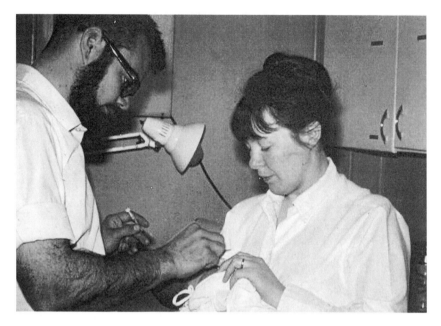

I vaccinate a baby while Muriel holds the patient—tightly!
FRANK DUNN PHOTO.

the south are not normally expected to do. One of these procedures involved taking X-rays and developing film. This meant learning the art of positioning the patient for the optimum picture of various parts of the anatomy. Since we were to be using what I thought was an ex-army Picker portable X-ray machine, we had to know how to limit the area to be filmed and how to use a lead apron, and we were given radiation monitoring badges that had to be worn whenever we used the equipment. The orientation even included how to mix the solutions for the developer and fixer and how to find our way around in the red glow of the safety lamp in the darkroom!

There was something of a medical controversy at that time about vaccines for TB, but government policy was that every man, woman and child who had a negative result to the TB test was to receive a Bacillus Calmette-Guérin (BCG) vaccination, which we were told would, or could, give 75 percent protection against the disease. (A negative result was determined when there was no local

114

skin reaction within three days after the antigen was injected under the skin.) Some doctors felt that, if the vaccination was given and the patient then had a positive skin reaction when tested, they would not know if it was a reaction to the vaccine or to a recent infection of the actual disease. However, we followed government policy and tested and then vaccinated all negative reactors including our own children. Dr. David Wilkinson, chief of the department of pediatrics at the Charles Camsell Hospital, had impressed upon us that we should not think of vaccinating any of the Native children until we had vaccinated our own, rather like "putting your money where your mouth is." We followed this advice with all the recommended vaccines that were available because we knew that vaccinations were effective and we wanted to protect our children.

After the X-ray survey was complete, we received the reports and charted them, then if there was suspicion of a small chest lesion in any of our patients, we had to try to get them to follow a preventive drug regime. I remember one old woman, well into her eighties, who was advised to take a huge number of TB pills every day, and as she was going out to her camp with her family for several weeks, I gave her enough pills to last her until she came back. I explained that taking them was very important, and she nodded and said, in the usual rather noncommittal Gwich'in way, "Aha, aha!" and took the plastic bag of pills from me. I visited her when she returned and she told me that she had taken the pills faithfully every day, but when I checked the bag I had given her, it was still full of pills. I don't think she had even opened the bag. In spite of this the old woman lived until she was 106!

In our six years of work in the nursing station we took hundreds of X-rays, mostly of chests, but also of heads, arms, hands, abdomens, legs and feet, and on more than one occasion we even X-rayed dogs. One elderly woman came into the clinic to have her foot X-rayed after she had fallen and thought that she had broken her toe. To aid in diagnosis we always X-rayed the uninjured foot so that we could compare them, but although this lady had taken off her mukluk for me to examine the injured foot, she was reluctant to remove the other one. I assumed that she was not prepared for this and perhaps had not washed the unaffected foot, but knowing that the X-ray would penetrate the moosehide without any difficulty, I placed both of her feet on the plate and took the shot, then went to the darkroom to develop it. The resulting picture was a bit perplexing because the good foot looked most peculiar and there was no fracture on the injured foot. I asked the lady what was wrong with her good foot and she looked a bit startled.

"What do you mean?" she said indignantly. "That foot is good!"

"Look at this," I said, holding up the still wet X-Ray plate for her to see. "It looks as though there are no toes on your right foot."

She glanced at the X-ray then at me and then at the floor. "I was born with this foot and the toes were all bent in. It was always like this but I manage okay. Even my old man doesn't know!" she said with a mischievous smile.

I told her that I wouldn't say anything to him about her club foot and she went home happily after I had taped up her injured toe. After that, whenever I saw her walking briskly on snowshoes or dancing on her toes at a community jigging dance, I was reminded of her adaptability. She would have been insulted if I had said that she had a handicap!

We were very surprised when Carol McCormack told us that current public health policies forbade her and the other nurses at the Health Centre from going out on emergency calls, which was certainly a change from when we had been the nurses there. Back in the sixties we had been told that patients should be expected to come or be brought to the nursing station for treatment, and this made sense because all the supplies and diagnostic equipment were available there. However, whenever we were called out by the RCMP—as happened when a young man was shot and seriously wounded one very cold winter's night—we went willingly to provide immediate care on site.

Another such emergency occurred one night when Muriel and I had gone curling, an activity that was new to us, but like some of the teachers from Outside, we were willing to try anything new. Although curling had long been popular in Scotland, I hadn't even heard of it when I had lived in England. The idea of sending a controlled "rock" down the ice to the centre of a painted circle seemed like a unique northern sport, so both Muriel and I signed up for the opening bonspiel after warning our skips that we had never seen a rock before. Besides, it seemed rather novel to go out at all times of the day and night—whenever our rinks' times came up— for a bonspiel, carry our corn brooms up to the log building that enclosed the one sheet of ice, and wearing our parkas, work up a sweat sweeping the ice. We quickly learned that the speed of the rock varied with the temperature outside; if it was thirty below outdoors, it was thirty below inside, and small ice flowers covered the ice sheet, making it almost impossible to get the rock to the end. If it was only minus five outside, the ice inside was slick, and if you used the same energy that you used on cold nights, the rock would go right through the other rocks, scattering them far and wide. The only problem with having both nurses curling at the same time—which sometimes happened even though we were on opposing teams—was that when an emergency occurred, our rinks were left short-handed. Of course, there were usually enough observers at the competitions that substitutes could be found, though it was difficult to find anyone with less or equal expertise than us.

It was in the middle of one of these bonspiels that William Firth appeared in the doorway and beckoned us over to him. "Mrs. Blake says that one of her grandchildren has been brought up from the Husky Channel because he has swallowed some lye."

Giving our apologies, we hurried down to the nursing station where we found the young boy and his mother in the waiting room. The mother did not know how much the boy had swallowed and only became aware that he had done it when he started crying because his mouth was sore. She had been using the lye on some skins and thought that there had been only a very small amount left in the container, but she had the foresight to give the young lad some re-constituted powdered milk to drink before bringing him up to the village. On examination we could see that his mouth was red and his lips looked puffy, but he had just been brought up the river on a dogsled and his face was red as well. Muriel and I conferred, and having decided that his breathing was okay and his mouth hadn't been too badly burned, we could wait for the regularly scheduled plane to send him to Inuvik.

"We won't take a chance that he hasn't burnt his throat, too," I told the mother, "so we are going to send him to Inuvik on the plane tomorrow and the staff there will be able to see down his throat and fix him up. Take him home to your mother's house and we will let you know what time the scheduled plane will be here. Don't give him anything to eat, maybe only sips of milk if you have to give him anything, and watch him carefully. Call us if you are worried, but he will be happier staying with you than he would be staying here."

With that the boy was bundled up and carried out. We made a note on his chart and wrote a letter to the doctor at the hospi-tal, then called it quits for the night. By now the bonspiel would be over and someone would tell us tomorrow who had won and whether or not we would be playing in the next round. We didn't hear anything from the family during the night. As soon as we were alerted to the plane's arrival time by the Pacific Western Air-lines agent, Alex Foreman, a Scotsman who also owned a store in town—he was referred to as a free trader, that is, a store other than the Hudson's Bay Company—we went to the house, checked on the young patient and arranged for the mother to accompany her son to the hospital.

About a week later we were happy to see the boy and his mother climb down from the plane. The doctor had found only slight burns to the throat and the boy was not expected to have any complica-tions from this misadventure. We were quite sure that the mother would now be very careful with chemicals, and she would be reminded time and time again of this incident by her own mother whom we knew to be very direct.

❋ ❋ ❋

Our work also included teaching public health, and it would have been impossible to do that sitting in the nursing station, although many Gwich'in people would remark that white people never visited the camps, as they had in the old days, to see if the Natives were doing okay. The white people, they said, did not want to go anywhere their machines couldn't take them and they liked to stay in their nice warm offices. Maybe that was true of a few who manned the nursing station or other government offices in Fort McPherson over the years, but it was also true that by the mid-nineties, when the Dempster Highway was in full use, not very many Gwich'in people went out into the bush for long periods of time either, and if they did go out to the mountains, they went on snowmobiles or in pickup trucks. Life had been very different when people travelled long distances by dogsled, and back then we felt that if we did not know how people lived in the bush, we could not advise them on good health practices.

Sometimes we received letters from people in the bush requesting medicine, though most often it was a demand for pain pills (Frosst 222s) or sometimes baby fever medicine. These letters were carried by anyone who was travelling up or down the Peel River, just as they carried parcels of dried fish, dried and fresh meat or any other piece of merchandise that was easily transported in a river boat or dog toboggan. But sometimes it was hard to tell from the letters exactly what was wrong or what was wanted, although fortunately the medical records that we kept sometimes helped us out. One old lady sent a letter that definitely made us wonder what her condition really was.

> *To Nurse in Charge.*
> *Dear Sir,*
> > *my compliment to you from hear is how I was this*

summer, I am still the same. I have no pain but really get pain in the evening All the remedies you sent me but no approvement in Day time I do my work but hope you sent me more pills or medicine

Thank you
Regard
Mrs XXX XXXX

This lady, who was in her eighties, lived in a cabin about one hundred kilometres up the Peel River. She had not gone there by taxi; she had driven a team of dogs, and when caribou or moose skins were brought to her she would work at cleaning and tanning the hides. She was mildly obese but still worked hard in the bush, handsawing and then splitting firewood before bending and lifting it to carry it to her cabin, a job hard enough even for young people. It was no wonder then that after she "did her work in the daytime" she really experienced pain in the evening. People of her age who lived in cities down south would be living in old folks' homes where there were no chores, and only easy chairs to sit in while they watched television and a comfortable bed at the end of the day. I was reminded of the old man who came to see a visiting doctor because he had a very painful back. This man spent the majority of his time living in a tent and sleeping on the floor, but the doctor told him to go home and put something firm under his mattress and he would feel better!

I sent the old lady a supply of 222s.

CHAPTER EIGHT

W HILE WE WERE VISITING IN FORT Mcpherson in 2009, a doctor arrived from Inuvik to hold a clinic for several days before going on to Tsiigehtchic to do another clinic; from there he would return to Inuvik via the Dempster Highway. We met with him very briefly after he arrived, but for most of our stay he was kept busy behind closed doors. I remembered reading a press release when the new hospital was built in Inuvik in April 2003, which had announced that there were seven doctors now on staff, and Ms. Praamsma, the assistant deputy minister of NWT's Health and Social Services, was quoted as saying that there were ten thousand people living in thirteen communities within the 1.5 million square kilometres the hospital serviced. I couldn't help but think back to those times when there had been no doctor in Inuvik at all and we had been left to our own devices.

But for Muriel and me, seeing this busy doctor at Fort Mcpherson was very reminiscent of the doctors' clinics held in our old nursing station. The doctor would fly into the settlement on the scheduled plane, usually arriving just before lunchtime, and the people, very aware that the doctor was there, would soon be packing into our small waiting room. After the clinic was over, usually well after ten at night, we would gather in the kitchen to relax with cups of tea or coffee. The doctor would usually sleep on the single bed in the maternity ward, but if a patient in labour was admitted during the night, we would have to turf him out of bed. This only happened once, and the visiting doctor was quite happy for Muriel to do the delivery as he happened to be an ophthalmologist. He apologized that though he was a doctor he was now more familiar with the other end of a patient.

I had spent the first few years of my professional life working in operating rooms, so as we sat over our cups of tea when the clinic was over for the day, I really enjoyed hearing stories about various procedures that the doctors had done, and I could briefly experience the exciting life in the operating room again. But for some reason—perhaps because we were all tired after the clinic—we would soon get to joking and laughing. One of the doctors, Dave Posen, regaled us with his life history, almost acting it all out, with his glasses pulled down his nose when he played the part of an old man, until Muriel and I were just rolling around. I was actually in pain from laughing but I didn't want him to stop, and even now, all these years later, whenever I remember his antics, I still want to laugh out loud!

Another doctor who visited us had been the personal physician and surgeon for his country's ruler, but while he was out of his country taking a course, that dignitary was deposed, and it had seemed unwise for the doctor to return to such a politically unstable country. Not having a licence to practice medicine in Canada, he took whatever work was available, even driving a cement truck, while he was getting the necessary papers to practice medicine here.

❄ ❄ ❄

On a few occasions, instead of the doctor coming to us in Fort McPherson, I took a patient to Inuvik and was able to participate in the procedures there. Early in 1965 a young Gwich'in man came to the nursing station complaining of a pain in his stomach. I asked the usual questions—where exactly does it hurt, for how long has it bothered you, questions about bowel habits and all of those other things that you wouldn't even tell your best friend. He mentioned that he had been throwing up "green stuff" for the past few days although he hadn't been eating.

When he had removed some of his clothes and indicated where his abdomen was hurting, I immediately thought: *Right lower quadrant, and all the symptoms pointing to appendicitis.* I then checked to see if there was any muscle guarding, which occurs when the overlying abdominal muscles become hard as though to protect the gut underneath. I also checked for rebound tenderness by pressing firmly on his abdomen then suddenly letting go. He winced.

"Did it hurt?" I asked.

"Not much," he said stoically.

I generally found that the Gwich'in men were very healthy. Their lifestyle included a high protein diet, mainly meat and fish, plenty of exercise as they ran for many kilometres behind their dog teams and good muscles from cutting, splitting and carrying firewood every day of their lives. As this young man's abdominal muscles were firm all over, I could not be sure about any particular guarding. A blood test would have told me more but we did not have the materials or capability to do blood work, which would have been a very helpful tool for this and other diagnoses. However, because of his symptoms, I was convinced that he did have appendicitis, and so I called Dr. Al Tajic at the Inuvik Hospital and discussed the case with him. Dr. Tajic was the most gregarious doctor we had met—friendly, a real social animal, and best of all, a very competent medical man and surgeon. He listened to the symptoms that I relayed to him over the phone, then told me to bring our patient to Inuvik by plane.

When we arrived at the hospital, I went with the patient to the examining room. Heidi Gunning, the X-ray technician, arrived with a portable machine, and I couldn't help seeing how much more sophisticated it was than our old ex-army Picker machine! She took an X-ray of my patient's abdomen and then a blood sample, and again I mourned our meagre supplies and equipment in Fort McPherson. Finally Dr. Tajic appeared, carrying the still wet X-ray sheet, which he stuck up on the viewing box, and flicked on the bright light. He shook my hand and I introduced him to the young man lying on the examining table. As I expected, Al went through the usual questions and examination, but I noticed that when he did the test for muscle guarding, he was much more aggressive than I had been. This time the young man brought his knees up and groaned.

"I'm inclined to agree with your diagnosis, Keith, although it is not a textbook case," Al said. "We'll wait for the blood sample results and then I will decide what to do." He turned to the patient. "We'll fix you up pretty soon. Just have patience with us."

When a nurse came in to do some routine work, blood pressure and temperature, we left and walked down to the hospital cafeteria for coffee. "You'll stay at our house tonight, Keith. I've already phoned my wife to let her know." His wife was a pediatrician who worked at the same hospital and they lived in a neat government house quite close by. When the lab report was delivered, Dr. Tajic remarked on the high white cell count, and then after a few moments said, "I think we will operate. Why don't you scrub in too, Keith? Then we'll both see what's inside!"

I was delighted at the prospect. I hadn't scrubbed up for an operation since leaving the Charles Camsell Hospital and that now seemed like another age. The operating room staff was advised of the impending surgery, another physician was called, and the young man that I had brought from Fort McPherson was wheeled into a room next to the operating room to be prepared. He lay there quietly, looking around, no doubt feeling nervous in this sparkling place that smelled of everything medical and where everyone walked around with masks covering their faces. Dr. Frank Bryce came in and explained that he would be putting him to sleep, but he would give him a shot first that would make him comfortable although it would make his mouth feel dry.

Dr. Tajic and I went into the scrub room where we stood side by side scrubbing our hands and arms for the required amount of time. Then, using sterile towels, we dried ourselves and put on the specially folded sterile gowns and masks, which were fastened up by the nurse who acted as the runner— the person who fetches and carries for the scrub nurse and the doctor. Then carefully donning sterile rubber gloves, we entered the operating room where the young patient was already on the table. Dr. Bryce was at the patient's head, half hidden behind a screen where the rhythmic sound of the anaesthetic machine could be heard as it automatically breathed for the unconscious patient.

I stood opposite Dr. Tajic and when sterile sheets were in place around the young man's abdomen and all was ready, he nodded to Dr. Bryce and the nurse handed him a scalpel. "I'm going to show you some really fancy surgery, Keith—keyhole surgery. We're going to do this job through a very small incision." He cut into the skin. "Catch those bleeders," he said as he continued working, and I picked up a curved artery forcep and clipped the small bleeding blood vessel, then went after another.

The incision was only large enough for Al to get his finger and thumb in, and when he reached the peritoneum, I thought it was going to be difficult. At this point all the instruments that had been used were considered "dirty," and to prevent contamination from the skin's surface, they were changed for fresh instruments—straighter and longer forceps and retractors. Al inserted his finger into the abdomen and hooked a piece of intestine, looking for the section where the small intestine joins the large intestine, a junction called the cecum, because it is here the vermiform appendix is found. After some poking around, he announced that he would have to enlarge the incision because he couldn't locate the appendix. Finally he said, "You're not going to believe this, Keith, but I think this lad has a very unusual gut. I have never come across this before. The appendix is on the other side, and I am going to have to make a new incision there!" I could see he was annoyed but mostly because he had wanted to show me some keyhole surgery. However, after conferring with Dr. Bryce and ascertaining that everything was okay at the anaesthetic end of the operation, adjustments were made to the green sheets that surrounded the operation site and Al started again on the left side of the abdomen.

Everything went well. He made an incision that was about ten centimetres long, and after a few minutes he located the appendix, removed it and in half an hour we were washing up and changing out of the OR greens into our street clothes. But Dr. Tajic couldn't get over what had happened. That night he related it all to his wife and the talk soon developed into a review of all the abnormalities they had experienced. After a very pleasant visit I left Inuvik the next morning and flew home. I had experienced a taste of the past, something medically different, and now I looked forward to being home in the present with my wife and daughter.

❅   ❅   ❅

It was also Dr. Tajic who made it possible for me to visit Old Crow in the Yukon. In the sixties it was one of the most isolated places in North America and consequently had retained a way of life that was fast disappearing from other northern villages. Like Fort McPherson, it had a nursing station, which the Inuvik doctors tried to visit on a monthly basis. Of course, it all depended upon the weather and the availability of doctors, and one month the job fell to Al Tajic, who flew first to Fort McPherson to hold a quick clinic before going on to Old Crow to hold one there. During a coffee break, he invited me to go along on the trip so I could have a quick look around while he held the clinic. He reassured Muriel that he would have me back home in Fort McPherson before dark.

After an early clinic we went down to the plane and I saw that Freddy Carmichael was using his Beechcraft for this trip. "When I fly over the mountains I like to have two engines," he said. Then he smiled and added, "Just in case!"

I had implicit faith in the northern pilots and their planes, and it had never occurred to me that the planes were not infallible. But of course, there are not many landing places for planes when you are up in the mountains! In later years I did hear of plane crashes, some where everyone survived and some where they did not. Martin Harwell had crashed when he apparently ran out of fuel after he became lost while flying to Yellowknife. On that trip three people died, including the nurse escort, but the pilot survived. In another instance,

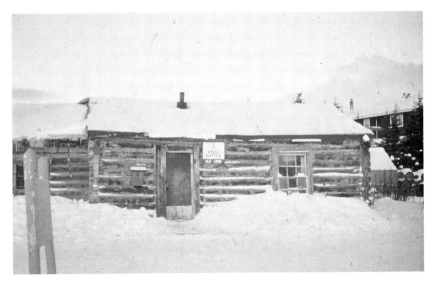

Although Old Crow, the nearest Gwich'in village to the west, was one of the most isolated places in North American, it still had a post office.

Tommy Gordon was flying a planeload of schoolchildren home to Fort McPherson from Inuvik in Freddy Carmichael's Beechcraft when both carburetors iced up and he had to make an emergency landing on a small lake. The snow was very deep and he brought the plane to a quick halt and everyone survived. After the children had all been ferried home in small planes, the Beechcraft had to be emptied of everything that wasn't essential, then the snow was cleared for the length of the lake and Freddy himself had to come down to fly his plane out.

One evening when we were listening to the radio station from Inuvik, an announcer broke into the regular programming with a special announcement. It was a message to a planeload of people who had been flying over the mountains from Alaska heading for Inuvik. Radio contact with them had been lost shortly after a mayday had been received. Although there had been no further communication and no sound from the emergency locator transmitter, the authorities were assuming that there were survivors and the message instructed them to light a fire so planes flying over could locate

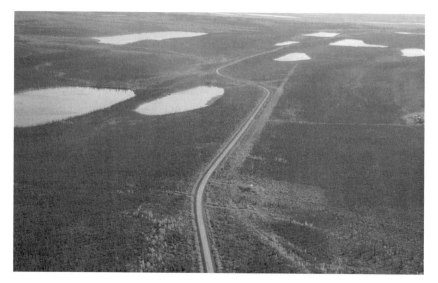

It's easy to get lost in the network of lakes and rivers in the Mackenzie Delta.

them. The message was broadcast every hour. I suppose privacy regulations prevented the radio station from doing a follow-up news item, but thankfully we had friends at the RCMP station who could pick up airplane communications, and the next day we learned that the plane had been equipped with all the latest electrical and communication systems but had experienced complete electrical failure. Fortunately, the pilot had managed to bring it down on a slope; there were no deaths and the only injury was one dislocated shoulder. An American helicopter managed to bring them all out safely.

With these memories in mind, I climbed into Freddy's Beechcraft, and we flew off over the foothills to the west of Fort McPherson and then over the Richardson Mountains toward Old Crow. I peered out the window, trying to see what route people would take to go overland between the villages, but we were flying too far south of the route that went from the Peel River, up the Rat River to the Yukon River via the Porcupine River.

We landed without incident in Old Crow and after a visit to the nursing station, I left Al Tajic and the nurse to go on with their

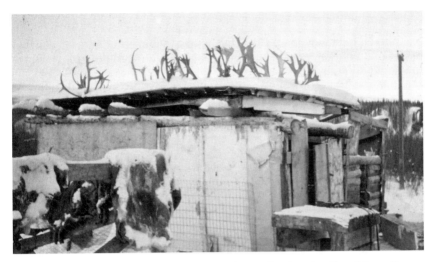

Caribou antlers on a meathouse in Old Crow display the Gwich'in reliance on caribou.

business while I made out like a tourist, visiting the post office and the new RCMP building before going to meet Edith Josie, a very typically quiet Gwich'in woman whose weekly column in the newspaper and on CBC National Radio had made her a well-known figure in the Arctic. The Old Crow people's dependence on caribou was obvious as I passed many of the small log buildings where dozens of antlers festooned the roofs.

All too soon it was time to return to the plane and we were soon on our way back to Fort McPherson. Below us the white mountains looked bare. I could see how easy it would be to get lost in them, as from the air each valley looked quite similar. I thought of the old days when the Gwich'in roamed these mountains, following the great caribou herds, and again I could not help but be impressed by these resourceful people.

❊ ❊ ❊

The traditional Gwich'in diet of dried meat, red meat, fish, berries and bannock was quite healthy, but I noted that they hardly ever ate vegetables, and although they seldom used sugar, they drank great quantities of tea and most had a daily tobacco intake. As a result, many of them suffered with dental cavities. A dentist would come to the village for a few weeks most years, but when he came, he worked almost exclusively on the schoolchildren. We did our best to squeeze in some of the adult patients for an evening clinic, but a lot depended on the dentist's forbearance.

One year, in an effort to give the few children who lived in Arctic Red River an opportunity to be seen by the visiting dentist, we talked Frank Bailey, the game warden, into bringing them to Fort McPherson. We knew he was going to be driving his big, tracked Bombardier to Arctic Red River over a seismic trail, though whether he actually got there would depend on the snow and ice conditions. These seismic roads had in recent years crisscrossed not only the Delta but most of the North as oil companies searched for subsurface deposits by releasing explosive charges at intervals of one-third of a mile. These winter roads or trails they constructed stretched straight as an arrow as far as the eye could see, and from the air the checkerboard pattern they made could be plainly seen. Frank was agreeable to bringing the children back with him but only if I would go along because, as he pointed out, "If the machine breaks down, I can't look after all those kids." Good point. Meanwhile, Al Jackson, the administrator at the school hostel in McPherson, agreed to have the children stay there overnight.

Frank and I set off early one morning, and if the vehicle had not had such good springs, I would have been jarred to death. I was not too surprised that when we were just over halfway there, the engine suddenly stopped. Frank fiddled around inside it and once more we were underway—for a short distance. Same thing again, stop, fiddle around, go again. This happened several more times. Finally he decided that there was a problem with either the gas or the carburetor, and when we got to Arctic Red River, he was going to order a new carburetor and filter and have them flown in.

I spent some time in the village deciding with the teacher which children should make the trip, but unfortunately, Frank had discovered that he couldn't get the parts he wanted. He was going to try to drive back to Fort McPherson, but he didn't want to take the children in case we ended up having to walk a long way. The children were disappointed at missing out on an adventure, but we all agreed it was the safest thing to do.

I would not be returning empty-handed, as I had been given several racks of stick fish, and then just as we were loading up, RCMP Corporal Don Rumple asked me if I could use a couple of beautiful two-month-old pups. When I asked why they wanted to get rid of them, he said that they were not sure of the sire, and as the RCMP had a dog breeding program, they could not keep them. Because the pups would have to travel inside the Bombardier cab with me, we put each one, with some difficulty, into a gunny sack. They made a lot of fuss until the engine was started, and then they just lay quietly in their sacks until we arrived home. The vehicle did not break down once and we made the trip in reasonable time. (The pups eventually became my lead and wheel dogs.)

※ ※ ※

Although the water supply for Fort McPherson was filtered and treated with chlorine, no fluoride was added so we were asked to provide a fluoride rinse for all the schoolchildren. This was not a problem for the teenagers in the more senior grades who had the self-control to hold the rinse in their mouths for the allotted time and then spit it out into waxed cups, which we then collected and disposed of. The young children, on the other hand, gave us and their teachers both a headache and a smile. We would carefully explain that they were to hold the cups with the "mouthwash" in their hands, then when I told them to, they were to put the liquid into their mouths and slosh it around. BUT THEY WERE NOT TO SWALLOW IT! Okay? They all nodded.

"Okay, put the stuff in your mouth now, AND DON'T DRINK IT DOWN!" For obvious reasons I was careful not to call the liquid a drink.

"Wash it around your mouth, hold it in your mouth. DON'T SWALLOW IT! Okay, now spit it out into the cup. DON'T SPILL IT!"

After the sounds of exaggerated spitting had filled the room, Muriel, the teacher and I went around to collect the cups. A quarter of them were empty, and most of those that had something in them got knocked onto the floor. Only a very few were successfully recovered. While it was a chore for us, the children thought it was a lot of fun!

Because of a shortage of dentists in the North, dental therapists were trained and hired to do some of the less complicated and preventative dental work, then because there was a shortage of dental therapists, the nurses in the settlements were left to do all emergency dental work. Fortunately, a part of the orientation that Muriel and I had received at the Charles Camsell Hospital was in the dental department, although in reality our whole dental orientation lasted just over an hour, after which we were expected to be able to do emergency fillings and extractions.

Perhaps because I was working in the operating room of the hospital and identification of instruments had become almost second nature to me, the dentistry program intrigued me. Of course, maybe I had just uncovered a latent sadistic characteristic. But Muriel did not feel comfortable doing this sort of work, and although she would do an extraction on an incisor if she thought she could grasp it well and the anaesthetic had worked, but when she saw a really bad molar, she would usually call me in.

The very first patient I saw needed a very bad lower molar removed. He had been suffering sleepless nights in agony, which is what it usually took before most of the men would come for treatment. I located my dental textbook and read the proper procedure for giving a dental block, where one whole side of the lower jaw is numbed with a local anaesthetic. I seated the patient on a wooden chair with a headrest clamped to the back of it, then turned the chair so that he had his back to the open cupboard in which I placed the book open to the appropriate page. Carefully following the steps in the book, I gave the injection and noticed with some relief that the patient still had his eyes closed. I waited and then saw him running his hand over his chin. "It feels funny," he said.

"Good!" I replied. "We'll leave it for a few more minutes."

I checked the gum around the tooth, and when the patient said that he couldn't feel anything, I picked up what looked like the right instrument and fitted it around the tooth. Remembering the mantra the dentist had told me at the Camsell Hospital, I told myself, "It's not brute strength that's needed. It's the action of the wrist that does the job!" By now the patient was perspiring and so was I, but with a quick movement out popped the tooth—to my surprise and the patient's relief! I gave him a piece of gauze to clamp over the wound, and as he got out of the chair, I hurriedly closed the cupboard door.

"That was really good!" he exclaimed through the gauze and his partly opened lips.

"No problem at all!" I lied.

Not all of my patients went away happy. One day when Muriel was seeing patients in the clinic and I was doing the usual charting and letter writing in the office close by, a young woman came in. I could hear the murmur of voices as she and Muriel spoke.

"Keith!" Muriel called from the clinic room. She didn't sound as though it was emergency but I put down the papers I was working on and went to the clinic. The patient was sitting in a chair looking very glum.

"Martha has a sore throat, and I think one of her teeth is causing an infection. Would you have a look to see if it should come out?"

Martha looked up at me and I nodded a greeting to her. "Let me have a look, Martha. Open your mouth wide so I can see where the bad tooth is."

As soon as she opened her mouth, she didn't have to point to the infected tooth. I could see what was left of it—just a crater surrounded by red tissue. There was no way it could be saved as there was nothing to fill.

I told Martha that I should take it out. "Is that okay?" I asked.

She didn't look too happy and glanced at Muriel before giving an almost imperceptible shake of her head. This I took to be agreement. I prepared the equipment I would need, shielding the instruments and the anaesthetic from the patient's view. I was going to have to give her a nerve block that would freeze the lower half of her jaw, and the needle I had to use was about five centimetres long. It was no good frightening her any more than she was already.

I placed her head in the headrest and told her I would give her a needle to deaden the tooth. I brought the needle up carefully so it would not be in her line of sight. Now, most patients close their eyes at this point, but Martha opened her eyes wide, caught sight of the needle, jumped up and pushed me away. "You're not going to stick that big needle in me!" she said, and she cowered as though I was going to attack her. I was glad that Muriel was still in the clinic room.

"That's okay," I said, although I was feeling a bit miffed at Martha's reaction. I had been looking forward to the challenge. "Muriel will give you some antibiotic, and it may help your throat, but someday that tooth will have to come out."

She just looked at me with wide eyes and I left her with Muriel.

By this time I was actually enjoying dental work because the patients were so quickly relieved of the terrible pain that brought them to the station. Unlike the case with Martha, I usually prevailed, though there was one case when the treatment was successful but my prognosis was wrong. A man who had been working on one of the exploration rigs was brought to the station in pain, and when I asked him what was wrong, he pointed wordlessly to his mouth. When he opened it, I saw that his gums were red and bleeding, swollen and infected, and his breath was foul-smelling. I immediately recognized an acute case of pyorrhea.

According to our dental book, his symptoms indicated that he could lose all of his teeth, and I told him this was a strong possibility because of the severity of his case. He told me that the company plane would be up in a day or two and he would be flown south, which I am sure was as much a relief to him as it certainly was to me. In the meantime, all I could offer him was a strong antibiotic. He was quite agreeable to this, so I gave him a large intramuscular injection of procaine penicillin, which was the best I could offer him at the time. I told him to buy a bottle of strong mouthwash at the store and use it frequently until the plane arrived to take him out. Then I wished him well, thinking that while he was outside, he would see a dentist and stay long enough to get some false teeth to replace the ones he was bound to lose.

It was almost a month later when the same patient walked in with a big smile on his face. "Remember me?" he asked.

He looked vaguely familiar but it wasn't until he pointed to his teeth that I remembered seeing him when he was so miserable with infected gums.

"They are all mine!" he said, continuing to smile as he told me that by the time the company plane delivered him to Calgary, his mouth was already healing. "That must have been a powerful shot," he said, adding that the dentist in the city had given him another shot but he didn't know what it was. I was glad to see a happy patient, though I felt humbled that I might have added to his early stress by telling him he would probably lose all of his teeth. But sometimes it was good to learn the hard way as long as our patients were not hurt in the process.

❄ ❄ ❄

From time to time an optician visited Fort McPherson to give a clinic, and on one such occasion, Old Martha, having heard on the radio that he was going to be in Fort McPherson, paddled down the river especially to see him. "Doc, I need new glasses." The old woman had skin like worn parchment, showing both her age and how weather-beaten she had become from a life facing the elements.

"What makes you think you need new glasses, Martha?" the doctor asked, taking her glasses from her and giving them a quick cleaning. He could see that the lenses were a bit scratched up.

"Sure, I need new glass. Few days back I shoot at caribou three times and that caribou he just run away!"

Martha had brought her rifle with her because she did not want to leave it in her canoe in case it was stolen. The doctor picked up the rifle and looked at it thoughtfully. It was an old model .303, quite scratched though well oiled, but we could both see that the barrel was attached to the stock with several turns of snare wire that had been covered with electrical tape.

"More likely you need a new gun, not new glasses!" he said.

"No, no, gun good, nothing wrong. Is my eye, he's no good!"

"Okay, I'll test your eyes and we'll see." He examined her eyes with his ophthalmoscope first and then with his optometric machine. He told me there was only a small change needed in her prescription and then he turned to her and said, "Martha, your eyes are pretty good, but I'll send you better glasses."

"Ah, good, good," she said, nodding gently. Getting up, she started to walk out then stopped, returned, bent down and picked up her rifle. "Good gun, this," she said knowingly to the doctor. "When that new glass come, I shoot that caribou!"

The doctor smiled and waved to her as she left the clinic. "I hope that when I'm her age, I can even lift a rifle, let alone go hunting!"

❄   ❄   ❄

Once a year the regional pharmacist would come to our nursing station to check our drugs and do an inventory of our medical supplies. We kept a register of all the narcotics used, with each patient's name and band number, the dose that we had prescribed and given, and a count of the narcotics left. Sometimes patients would describe their symptoms to us and then ask for pills to cure them of whatever they thought they had. However, we had to get a good history and maybe do more investigations before prescribing, which they probably considered a waste of time. Unfortunately, we did not have a different pill available for every disease that was in the book. Once rather facetiously we told the pharmacist that we should be issued with a supply of placebos because people were always demanding pain pills and we were reluctant to give out too many at any one time.

While the pharmacist was visiting, we would also invite the RCMP officer-in-charge to come round and check the narcotics, and when Jim Simpson was the corporal, he would relieve the boredom of counting thousands of pills by making jokes as he was counting. Using a pill-counting tray, he would start counting and then when he reached somewhere around seven hundred of the tiny phenobarbital tablets he would look up with a mischievous smile and say, "Now was that 702 or 712?" Then with a shrug he would carry on counting, leaving us wondering if our count was going to come out the same.

I don't think he considered it an important job because he knew that if we were satisfied and the pharmacist was satisfied and the records were in order, he would be satisfied, too.

Demerol, phenobarb, morphine and a host of other controlled drugs were all counted and recounted, then old pills or surplus pills were separated out and either flushed down the toilet or burned, all under the watchful eye of the corporal who didn't mind this chore as long as he had a cup of coffee in one hand.

CHAPTER EIGHT

IT WAS THE WHITE MAN WHO first brought alcohol into Gwich'in communities and it created a never-satisfied thirst for most of the people who tried it. Home brew, which was quite legal if a permit had been obtained from the RCMP, was the most commonly used intoxicant in Fort McPherson, and though it was not very potent, it was used in large quantities so the effects were the same as if it had been strong liquor. However, it was not the alcohol itself that was the problem in most cases but what happened within the families as the direct result of the drinking. Wives and children were abused; children were left cowering in corners when their fathers beat their mothers, who in turn shouted obscenities. Families that used to be friends would now be at each other's throats, people who had steady jobs lost them because they didn't show up for work after a binge, and those who were known to drink frequently were never even hired.

In a study published in 1963, Donald Clairemont[2] described two patterns of drinking among Delta residents: the splurge and the one-night bout. The first occurred after all the liquor in the village had been drunk and no one had the money to charter a plane to Inuvik to buy more. Then, when money became available from the selling of furs or perhaps a paycheque, the recipient flew to Inuvik where he stayed until the money and the liquor ran out. This individual would then prowl around looking for something to drink—mouthwash, aftershave lotion, vanilla extract, anything that may contain alcohol. The one-night bout was the result of several people in the village pooling their resources to cover the cost of sending a reliable person to Inuvik to bring home liquor, after which a "planned" party took place. Usually people who had some responsibility in the community used this pattern of drinking. Clairemont summarized his findings by stating that one of the functions of alcohol is to help people overcome shyness and to permit easy interaction among people at events where large numbers are present, although it is also used as a symbol of friendship. In later years it became apparent that some of the alcohol abuse was caused by conflict within the age group that either grew up in residential schools away from parental influences or were brought up in a "white world" without many of the benefits of that world.

Of course, Clairemont wrote his report before the Dempster Highway was built, and now that it provides easy access between communities, we wondered about the present situation. People had told us that there was still "quite a problem" in the settlements with alcohol and drugs, but in 2009, as we drove around the Mackenzie Delta, we were hardly aware of such problems. Of course, we didn't frequent places where we could be expected to see intoxicated persons, so we were spared this sad spectacle.

Back in the sixties the police had dealt with those who got into trouble because of excessive drinking, and they had usually brought their charges to us when there was a medical problem involved. Late one night Constable Mel Peletier brought in a young woman who was so intoxicated she could hardly stand up. She had been severely beaten and her eyes were both swollen shut, her nose was a bloody pulpy mass and her lips were swollen and disfigured. Mel asked if I knew who she was, but I couldn't recognize her facial characteristics at all, and perhaps because she was in police custody, she wouldn't say a word to me or to the police. We called Muriel in, but she was at a loss to identify her as well, and after she had examined her, we told Mel that her tissues were so swollen that it would be impossible to put any sutures into her wounds. We would reassess the situation the next day if he would bring her down to the nursing station again. Muriel cleaned her up and she left wordlessly with the constable.

The next morning Mel called to say that they were releasing the woman and she did not want to come to the clinic. Then he added that someone had identified her for them and he mentioned her name. I couldn't believe what I heard. The woman in question was only in her early twenties and she was (or had been) the most beautiful girl in the village. I could only wonder what she had done to have an assailant damage her face so badly, but what came to both our minds was that she had made someone very jealous at a party and had suffered the consequences. Because she would not identify her assailant, the RCMP could not lay charges.

❉ ❉ ❉

In a few special cases we were taken to the problem. I recall one case where a woman in her twenties had gone to an oil exploration base camp on the west side of the frozen Peel River opposite the village, walking there over a hard-packed snowy trail. She had evidently been successful in her quest for alcohol and had decided to walk back in the middle of the night. It was only a short distance from the camp to the village—in fact, she must have seen the village lights from the camp—so she had followed the trail down the hill from the camp and then, probably because of her confused state of mind, left the trail in an attempt to walk in a straight line toward the village lights. Once off the trail she had floundered in the undisturbed snow, which was deep, loose and fluffy because there were willows growing in that area and the wind had not packed it down. She had become tired and must have lain down in the snow to rest, and that is where she stayed until a man setting out with his dogs early the next morning to get firewood had seen a dark object lying in the snow. Stopping to investigate, he found that she had frozen to death.

When the RCMP officer came to get us, he said there was no doubt that the young woman was dead as her limbs were frozen, but one of us had to see her to certify that she was indeed dead. "And we want you to try to get a blood sample from her so we can determine if she has consumed alcohol and, if so, how much." When I saw the body, it was surrounded by footprints, and the police had already mapped out her uncertain progress from the camp across the river. Purely out of habit, I tried to obtain some blood from the victim's arm but it was so frozen that it was impossible. Now my only hope of obtaining any sort of sample would be from the heart and I decided to try this as her trunk appeared to be less solidly frozen than her limbs. Pushing a needle deep into someone's chest is not for the squeamish, and I thought that I was hardened to such things, but it took a deep breath and a great deal of resolve not to show my hesitation while others were looking on as I positioned a long needle on the 20cc syringe and pushed it into the frozen flesh. I managed to obtain a syringe full of blood, which I handed over to one of the officers, and I was very glad to be finished with that part of the operation. The young woman's body was then taken to the nursing station to be kept there until thawed enough for us to prepare her properly and then place her in a coffin.

After sad and miserable jobs like this, Muriel and I would sit down to talk about the Gwich'in people and their lot in life. We could understand the frustration of the young people, living in a world where they were being educated and prepared for—what? They did not have the confidence to leave the village and go out into the world, but if they stayed in the village what was there to look forward to? Unfortunately, we did not have a crystal ball to gaze into or we would have seen that some of these Gwich'in youngsters would go on to get a higher education and return to their community to become leaders, professionals and administrators.

❅ ❅ ❅

But it wasn't only the young people who suffered the consequences of heavy partying. One afternoon we got a message to call at the house of Mrs. Patrick because she had hurt her leg and couldn't walk. As Muriel and I were on our way through the village anyway,

141

we agreed to stop and check on her and then if necessary get a ride for her down to the nursing station. Mr. Patrick ushered us into a dark and dismal house and pointed to his wife who was sitting up on the side of their bed. "She hurt her leg about three days ago but it isn't getting any better."

We pulled back the blanket and saw that as she sat on the side of the bed, her left leg stuck out at a right angle to her trunk.

"I think her hip is broken," I said quietly to Muriel.

"Why didn't you send for us when this happened?" Muriel asked, meanwhile gently probing the top of the hip with her fingers.

There was no immediate answer then her husband said apologetically, "We were having a party and she must have fallen, and she didn't want me to call you in case you'd be mad at her for drinking."

"We will have to take her to the nursing station to X-ray her hip and then, by the look of it, she will probably have to go to Inuvik." Then Muriel turned back to Mrs. Patrick and said, "It must be very painful."

"It hurts when I move, but it's not too bad." But she winced even as we put the blanket around her again.

Once again we commandeered the police truck, and after collecting a stretcher from the nursing station, we returned to the Patrick house. With the constable's help, we gently moved the injured leg until it was parallel to her good leg then applied a special splint to the injured leg. When this was complete, we were able to lift her onto the stretcher, and the constable and Mr Patrick carried her out to the truck. Once we had her in the nursing station and moved onto a hospital bed, I trundled our Picker portable X-ray machine over and took a picture of the hip. In the darkroom I immersed the film in the developing liquid. To me this process was always like magic, and as the film started to develop, I kept lifting it out to see what was happening. The femur began to appear and then the hip joint and when at last the film was ready, I was able to lift it right out, rinse it off and hold it up against the red safety light. And there it was! The neck of the femur was completely broken off. I hurriedly put the film into the fixer solution, and after waiting a few minutes I was able to carry the still dripping film to the clinic where we had a lighted film holder. Muriel gazed at it, shaking her head. "I can't imagine sitting up with that for three days! She must have been in agony!"

When I phoned the hospital for a medevac, the doctor asked, "You're sure it's broken, Keith?"

"Oh, there's no doubt about it. The head of the femur is broken right off at the neck. It's going to need pinning." Then realizing I was talking to a doctor, I added, "I think."

It was still light when the plane arrived, and with the same help that we'd had earlier, we took Mrs. Patrick to the plane, loaded her in and she was whisked away to hospital, accompanied by a nurse who had come from Inuvik. Sure enough, the bone had to be pinned, but Mrs. Patrick returned to Fort McPherson within a very short time and we visited her at her home. She had a very stiff hip but said she had no real pain, and she was managing to move around the house with the aid of a crutch that the hospital had given her.

"Next time," I said, hoping there wouldn't be one, "please let us know when you are hurt. We won't bite your head off, you know." Then I added, trying to be humorous, "Well, not too badly anyway."

She looked up at me without a smile and said the non-committal, "Aha."

I left the house.

✳   ✳   ✳

One New Year when we had been hoping for a peaceful holiday, our hopes were shattered when the incoming year was barely an hour old. When our doorbell rang, I made my way to the clinic door with bleary eyes. The cold that wrapped its fingers around my bare legs and face when I opened the door soon took the sleep out of my eyes, and then seeing Frank, the RCMP constable standing in the doorway, my mind went on full alert within seconds.

"Come on in," I said, trying not to shiver as I spoke. "It's cold!"

"We need you at the school hostel, Keith," he said, stepping inside. "Floyd Worthington is in a bad way. Someone found him on the floor in the boys' washroom. I don't know if he's alive."

This was not the sort of information I wanted to hear at this hour of the night, but that was why we were here and I rushed to the bedroom to get dressed. It was fifteen minutes later when we drove up to the hostel in the police truck, and Frank immediately led me to the washroom upstairs.

The staff of Fleming Hall, the Anglican hostel for the schoolchildren, were very busy people when school was in because it was a big responsibility to look after all these young children, but they were all confident and gentle people and the children seemed to respect them. They were overseen by Al Jackson, the administrator, a very quiet but firm, middle-aged man who was well respected by parents and children alike. The hostel was divided into two wings with the girls' dormitory on the second floor of the west wing and the boys' in the east wing, each with a large washroom close by. The staff rooms and a small clinic room were located between the dorms. On the main floor were classrooms, where the children did their homework, the dining area and kitchen and the administration office.

Muriel and I didn't know very much about the boys' supervisor at Fleming Hall, Floyd Worthington, except that he had also been appointed a justice of the peace, so when infractions of the law were brought to his attention by the RCMP, he would hold court and mete out appropriate justice. All serious cases would, of course, be referred to a higher court. We sometimes saw him out on local trails with his Boy Scout troop but we rarely saw him down at the clinic unless he brought one of the boys in his care to us for treatment. Unfortunately, he was one of those people who, when invited to a house party, became very morose after he had one or two drinks, but apart from being a bit of a bore at Christmas parties, he was never a problem.

Now as we entered the washroom, I could see that the corporal had been taking photographs and making notes while he waited for us. "Hi, Keith," he said, stepping away from the prone figure at his feet. "This is a bit of a mess, isn't it?"

"Fortunately there are no kids in the hostel tonight," Frank said.

"It would have been tough on one of those little tykes if they had walked in on this."

Floyd was lying on his back on the hard terrazzo floor. I felt for a pulse and, finding none, checked his chest with my stethoscope. Nothing. His eyes were open and he was not breathing. I asked how long ago he had been found and was told that it was nearly an hour earlier. I told the officers there was no doubt that he was dead, but these men were used to unusual and tragic events and casually accepted the fact that they would now have to investigate the cause of his death.

"We know he was drinking a lot last night," Frank said, "because we saw him earlier and told him that he should come back here— which he must have done. What complicates this is that he is a justice of the peace and we have to make sure no one took advantage of him for some kind of revenge."

We looked around but there was no sign of a struggle and the position of the body suggested that he had fallen over backwards from the sink, perhaps striking his head on the hard flooring.

But why had he fallen? Had he fainted? The sink, which was directly in front of where he lay, was stained with blood and what looked like saliva. My guess was that he had felt nauseated, came to the sink to vomit, saw the blood he was expelling and passed out, falling backwards and striking his head on the floor. Some bloodstains on the countertop around the sink suggested that he may have wiped his mouth as he stood there, and then as he fell backwards his hand had smeared the blood on the countertop. When I examined his left hand, sure enough, there were blood stains there. There was nothing else I could do for Floyd now. Everything else was police work.

"Because of who he is, we will have to get an autopsy done," the corporal said. "You never know if someone put some ground glass in his drink or something way out like that. We'll have to call the police plane in tomorrow. Frank, will you run Keith home in the truck? I'll stay here and finish making notes until you get back."

The procedure that the corporal had suggested sounded a bit sophisticated for a quiet Gwich'in village, but I was glad this was now in the RCMP's hands because they would take care of the body and they would have to find and notify the next of kin. However, I couldn't just put the event out of my mind and go home to bed again. Floyd had been someone we knew, even though slightly, and I wondered what effect his death would have on the community members who, I was sure, expected the white people to be above anything sinister. So I declined the ride back to the clinic, thinking that a walk in the cold night air would clear my head a bit. I was halfway through the village when a man lurched from between two cabins. "Hey, Keith!" he called drunkenly, "my stomach is really bothering me." William Charlie was normally a pleasant man but I had no time for someone who was drunk and expected a miracle cure in the middle of the night.

"Look," I said exasperatedly, "if you didn't drink so much, you wouldn't have a bad stomach. I've got no sympathy for you, especially tonight. So go home and get some sleep and come and see me in the clinic when you're sober." I turned and went on toward the clinic, leaving William standing there in the street. I soon forgot the incident, but strangely enough he reminded me of it when I met him again forty years later. He thanked me with a laugh and no sign of rancor and said that after my tough talk he had gone home and had been sober ever since!

When I got back to the nursing station after Floyd's death, I sat down in the office, all thought of sleep gone, and made some notes because I knew from past experience that any cases involving the police usually required some official notes. It was months before we heard that nothing untoward had been found at Floyd's autopsy, apart from a severe gastric alcohol-induced hemorrhage, but no ground glass or poisons, and I guess we were relieved that no one else had been implicated in his death. His body was flown south where his relatives took care of the funeral arrangements.

CHAPTER TEN

I N THE PAST MOST PUBLIC SERVANTS and those people from Outside who had come North to do a specific job stayed only as long as their contracts demanded, but Muriel and I quickly noted that it was those Outsiders who did not participate in community activities or were not adventurous who usually did not like living in the North. Some of them had only come, it seemed, to make money, and they went to work day by day and otherwise stayed home. The women were usually only there because of their menfolk and most did not have jobs to go to, so they stayed home with or without children, and as the dark winter months dragged on, all sorts of problems developed. Sometimes we had to act as marriage counselors and would find ourselves at a loss about what to say when some woman would tell us a tale of woe and say, "You understand, don't you?" I guess we really did understand, but it was sometimes tempting to tell couples to get out into the fresh air and mix with the local people and then perhaps they would have a different perspective on life. For people who missed window-shopping or the social life at the local pub in the city, there was no easy answer except to look for work down south.

The whole question of mental health in the North had been addressed in an official report back in 1959 when it asked:

How long should the average Canadian, brought from the South to the North to work, stay there on a single tour of duty?

Is the Canadian who is willing to work in the North "average"
in the first place? Can he be persuaded that the North presents
a wonderful challenge, which makes it worthwhile living in a
large wooden box perched amidst a vast bleak waste, minus the
recreational facilities which in the South he takes for granted?
Should his wife and children accompany him and if so, how
can she be kept happy and they be given the opportunities for
growth and development that most Canadians take for grant-
ed? What makes a man "bushed"; just what is this condition
and how can it be prevented?[3]

In our experience, the people from Outside, sometimes called transients, stayed for varying amounts of time. Schoolteachers stayed an average of two years, whereas the game wardens and the Indian agents we met had all spent a long time in the North but only stayed in one settlement for about two years. The engineers and electricians who looked after the Northern Canada Power Commission (NCPC) generators varied widely in the time they spent in a village. The NCPC superintendent usually stayed longer than the others, but this operation also hired some of the local Gwich'in men who, of course, lived in the village and worked there for a number of years. The Fleming Hall hostel staff were employees of the government but seemed to be affiliated with the church and stayed in the community for much longer periods of time than the average Outsider. Then there was the nursing staff who came for periods of from one to two years. When we were sent North, we had to commit to spending two years or pay a percentage of our travel costs back to the government. We said that we would stay for two years and ended up staying for six, which was almost unprecedented then, although Carol McCormack, the incumbent nurse in charge in Fort McPherson, has already been there with her daughter for nine years.

RCMP officers rotated on a two-year basis. In those days the police had to apply for northern duty and they could be sent to the Yukon or the eastern or western Arctic, but as far as I could find out,

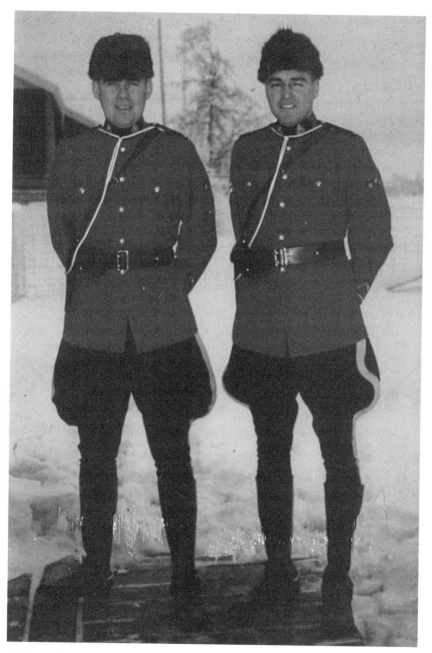

Officers Constable Frank Dunn and Corporal Shane Hennan. RCMP of-ficers rotated on a two-year basis, and in our experience, public servants stayed only as long as their contracts demanded.

they all seemed to enjoy their postings because it was what they had asked for. But when one of the popular young Mounties had not been seen around the village for quite some time, we wondered if he had been unhappy in his posting and asked if he had been transferred. The corporal's answer was a simple "No" without any further elaboration, so we assumed he must be on an extended holiday. However, this young officer had actually gone undercover in Yellowknife in an attempt to break into a drug and alcohol gang. After it was all over we heard that he had gone unshaven for weeks, worn old clothes and generally looked a mess as he frequented bars and managed to gain the confidence of the people he was investigating.

Everything was going well for him until one night he was sitting in a Yellowknife bar with members of the gang and was just getting to the point where he could learn some important facts about the case when the Gwich'in chief from Fort McPherson came into the bar and did a double take when he spied the young officer sitting with a bunch of ruffians.

"Hey, John!" he called out. "How ya doing? I haven't seen you for a long time. You still in the Force?"

The young officer jumped up from the table, hooked his arm into the chief's and quickly took him outside. He explained that he had been working undercover for weeks and now his cover had been blown by the one in a million chance that someone who knew him as an officer in the RCMP had recognized him. Of course, it could have happened if he had been in Edmonton or Calgary, and he was able to laugh about it later, but he told us afterwards that he had been put in a very dangerous position.

The Mental Health Report cited above also stated:

The efficiency of an employee in a small northern settlement is cut down by the percentage of his time that must be spent in living. If he is overambitious or tries to "build Rome in a day," he may be greatly frustrated by the time that must be used in servicing power plants, checking supplies, making out requisitions, keeping records, preventing food from freezing or thawing, changing stove parts, caulking windows, cleaning chimneys, filling in forms, etc. but it all tends to build an amount of patience that is intolerable to southerners; adaptability is strengthened.

❋ ❋ ❋

Nursing station activities kept both Muriel and me busy most of the time, especially in the dark days of winter when, as could be expected, aches and pains, colds and coughs were rampant and, in a close-knit community, spread quickly from one to another. Thankfully there were also very quiet periods, especially when the bright sunny days of spring made everyone feel generally healthy. It was at times like this that I enjoyed doing maintenance work on the station building. It had been prefabricated and brought down the Mackenzie River by barge twenty years previously and was now looking a bit shabby. Its shingled walls had been painted a beige colour with the standard northern red shingle roof, but our request to have it repainted went unanswered. Instead, we heard some vague references to the construction of a new station "in a few years."

One spring as the snow melted and we were again struggling through mud as we made our rounds, we found very few people at home, and I came back to the station and took a good long look at our building. To my biased eye, it was the colour of mud, and I went inside to discuss painting it with Muriel. William Firth was still the janitor and handyman at that time, and the station was his pride and joy, but he was getting older and frail and I did not want to ask him to go climbing ladders and risk being injured. But if I did the job myself, I risked incurring his wrath because, like most people in their seventies, he felt fit and would not want a young upstart to think he couldn't do the job.

When we next sat down for a coffee break with William, I started complaining about how quiet it was and how it would stay that way until after breakup. I told him that I was bored and was even thinking that putting some paint on the building would give me something to do and would freshen up the place a bit. He considered this information for awhile and then said that it was a good idea. "But if you need any help just call me and I'll come and do it."

With that settled, I went whining to our friends at the RCMP barracks and then to the Indian agent looking for paint handouts. The police had gallons of white paint, which they used for their buildings. They even painted the rocks that marked out their pathways. Les, the Indian agent, had some turquoise blue that would make a good contrasting trim on the building. The weather forecast was for warm and dry over the next few days, so as soon as the sun had warmed the air the next morning, I changed into some old coveralls, hoisted up a ladder and got to work.

The second day, while Muriel went to the village to check up on one of the old ladies, I worked my way to the peak at the south end of the building, heartily daubing white paint on the shingles. It was at that point that the law of probability came into play, and a man came down the road holding out his arm and hollering, "Keith, I've hurt my arm! Can you help me?"

Now what was I going to say to him—"Sorry, but I'm enjoying painting?" Of course, the government did not employ me to paint its buildings, and even if it had, I would have felt a moral obligation to provide help to anyone who required it.

"Of course, I'll come right down!" I called and hustled down the ladder, took off my coveralls, and went inside to see the patient who was now waiting at the clinic door. It was at that point that I saw my hands were covered in paint. Then inspiration came to me. I quickly went into the clinic room and pulled on a pair of brown latex examining gloves, hoping the paint would not dry and stick the rubber to my skin or to the hairs on the back of my hands. I was now ready to examine the patient's arm as he explained that he had been up a ladder, and instead of moving it, he had reached over for something that was too far away. As he fell to the ground, the ladder had landed on his outstretched arm. This kind of fall will often cause a break of the wrist called a Colles' fracture, but when I felt down his forearm, I didn't think it was broken. To make sure, I took an X-ray and it confirmed that the bones were intact and he had only sustained a bad sprain. I put his arm in a sling and sent him off after telling him to be more careful when he next went up a ladder.

I donned my coveralls again and went back to my painting job, and as I ascended the ladder, I thought how easy it was to be over-confident. It would only take one wrong step or overreach and I could be lying in the garden waiting for Muriel to come home. But I finished painting the walls and then the trim without any incident, thoroughly enjoying the project. However, I was glad that I had seen the patient with the sprained wrist, because it had made me so much more conscious of how accidents could happen.

Dr. Boag, in an article in the *American Journal of Psychiatry*, had noted that many people who went north were not motivated to "make a go of it," and he said that their non-verbal behaviour showed the following characteristics:

> *Apathy, lack of interest in their surroundings, greatly increased hours of sleep, lack of attention to personal appearance and tidiness of quarters and disinclination to undertake extra work or odd jobs in spite of complaints of not having enough to do. Men would frequently start the [year] with extensive plans for spare time activities, only to fail almost completely in carrying them out.*[4]

I knew that neither Muriel nor I fitted into this category, but when I read the report, I did note the sentence about "lack of attention to personal appearance" and I began to wonder at what stage I was in. Of course, we would normally only appear in public after showering and dressing appropriately, but there are always those times when "appropriate" could give the wrong impression.

One summer we were asked if we minded riding herd on a half-dozen senior medical students from Quebec who were to spend a few weeks in Fort McPherson. The idea was for them to gain some rural experience, and I am sure someone in the federal government also thought that this would serve as a recruitment ploy. The six male students arrived by float plane, and we soon found that, besides being interested in medicine, they also had a desire to know about the Gwich'in people. But what was disturbing to us, especially not knowing about it beforehand, was the fact that a magazine reporter accompanied them to document their experiences with both camera and notebook. We also discovered that although the students were indeed interning doctors, they had little or no experience outside of a hospital—and with some of them we were soon wondering what experience they had inside a hospital! This was after we noticed one of them trying to draw some pediatric oral penicillin into a syringe. However, they were all outgoing and it was fun taking them with us on home visits, and most of our elderly patients enjoyed having the young docs fuss over them.

The subject of appropriate dress came up during their visit because it was my habit to go very early in the mornings down to the river where I had moored a scow, and then casting off, motor downriver a short way to where I had set a net from which I collected enough fish to feed my dog team for the day. My early morning trip was detected, because I returned in my old clothes, probably smelling of fish, with a toque pulled down over my ears because it was cold on the river. Naturally, this presented a fine photo opportunity for the reporter, who asked me to take him and a couple of the interns with me one morning. I warned them that it would be cold, and they arrived at the boat dressed warmly, but unlike me they were all neatly dressed. Oh well, I had to get fish for the dogs so away we went, the reporter's camera at the ready. I hauled in a good supply of fish, which was all duly recorded on film, but all I could think about was that the government was onto a good thing recruiting doctors, and if these photographs of the local nurse dressed like a bum and fishing for breakfast ever got published, recruitment for nurses would be dismal.

We then organized a trip by boat to Arctic Red River so the interns could see the people and the village. As my boat was too small, I talked Don Wootten, the Anglican minister, into renting us his boat, which had a cabin. Don had never been to Arctic Red River so I suggested that he come, too, and he could captain his own boat. We loaded several barrels of gas into the stern, and on the appointed day we set off. Everyone enjoyed the scenery and meeting a few people at the Mouth of the Peel village, and our visitors were suitably impressed by the size and volume of water that flowed down the Mackenzie River. The only excitement I had was when I noticed one of the interns sitting in the stern and using the top of a full forty-five gallon barrel of gas for an ashtray!

We stayed a short time in Arctic Red River and then set off down the Mackenzie for Inuvik, but we hadn't gone very far when Don reported that the boat was very sluggish, and when we went into the cabin, we found water up to the gunwales and coming in fast. A quick turnaround soon had us back in Arctic Red River, where Dale Clark came to our rescue. Pulling the boat up the riverbank so the bow was out of the water, he discovered a hole in the bottom and guessed that we had hit a submerged log. A small piece of plywood, some adhesive and a dozen nails soon made a good patch to cover the hole from the inside, and we were once more on our way. Again, I was impressed how most of the Gwich'in people could make running repairs to nearly anything, using whatever was at hand, and if they hadn't got a suitable part, they would try making one. One man was reported to have made a part for an outboard motor water pump out of a carved piece of bone from a moose's shoulder blade.

Apart from hitting a rock and breaking the cotter pin in the middle of the channel that led to Inuvik, we arrived there safely and enjoyed a meal at the hospital before heading back to Fort McPherson. We were windblown and tired, but I think the young interns returned to Quebec having had some good experiences in the Mackenzie Delta.

CHAPTER ELEVEN

Ⅰ N THE ARCTIC THE SUN DOES not rise at all between early December and early January and during that time Fort Mc-Pherson experiences its coldest temperatures. The nursing station thermometer would go down to somewhere below minus sixty degrees (C), almost at the bottom of the gauge, and when we peeked outside we could see smoke from all the blazing wood stoves hanging over the village like a blanket. Then on January 6 the faintest tip of the sun would show over the southern horizon, and it was enough for us all to know that good weather would soon be with us. Not good weather where we could go around in shorts and tee shirts, but good weather that would give us relatively warm sunny days, which when travelling over the tundra or the lakes with a good dog team could lift a person's spirits and make him or her want to sing out loud—or at least that is how it affected me!

❊ ❊ ❊

Teachers, the police and their families and others from Outside would get together in someone's house to hold a "sun returning party," and we would try not to remember that we still had four and a half months or more of snow ahead. Of course, I am sure the Gwich'in people thought that the long dark nights had finally got to us! Muriel and I would go the host's house carrying our medical bags in case we were called out. William and Mary always knew

156

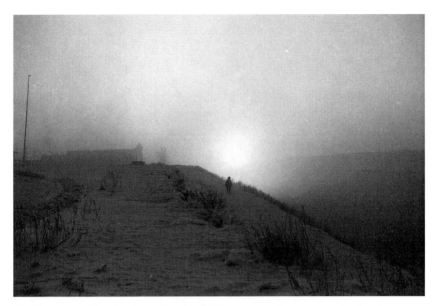

On January 6th, the first glimpse of the sun peeking over the horizon was enough to assure us that good weather was on its way.

where we could be found, but I also felt sure that there would not be many villagers who didn't know where the activity was.

Perhaps it was those long winters or the isolation that drove me to do some crazy things in the North, though at the time I thought I was just satisfying my curiosity and wondered why no one else had tried to do some of these things. One day I was out on the frozen Peel River and, noticing that there was a long stretch of smooth ice covered with only about half a metre of snow, I wondered what it would be like to ski on it. The trouble was that the temperature was minus twenty-five and regular ski boots would soon freeze the feet off anyone crazy enough to wear them. On the other hand, wearing mukluks is not conducive to fitting your feet into any manufactured boot or ski. Then I remembered that my old water skis were sitting in the shed up at the nursing station. I had brought them north with me because I didn't have a clue what to expect, and so on a whim I had thrown them in with other things that were being packed to be sent to Fort McPherson. They were made of laminated wood

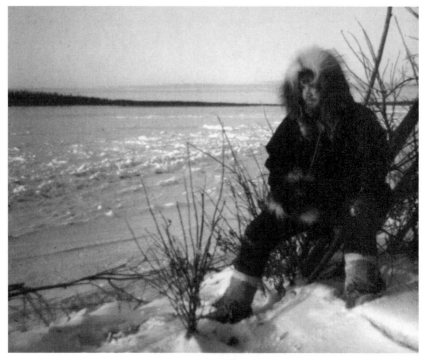

Looking over the Peel River is an opportunity to contemplate life in the North.

with a gentle curve at the front and were about twenty-two centimetres broad.

When I arrived home that day, I dug out the skis and was pleased to see that the foot piece was big enough to insert my foot into it while wearing mukluks. My next job was to organize some form of power to move me across the snow. If a speedboat would work in water in the summertime, why not a snowmobile in the wintertime? So I recruited Walter Alexie's snowmobile and Dave Sullivan, the Bay manager, volunteered to drive it. I also needed a tow rope and settled for a length of rope with a loop at one end to grip. I didn't want to be in a position where the rope could snag me and drag me along, as snow and ice are far less forgiving than water. As soon as we had everything ready, we drove down to the river and I prepared for "the ride of my life."

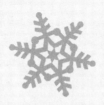

Winter could bring warm chinook winds, raising the temperature by thirty or forty degrees in a matter of hours, making travel by dogsled virtually impossible. Then usually within forty-eight hours the winds would change again and extremely cold weather would result.

In a bulletin that Richard Slobodin wrote for the National Museum of Canada about the weather in the Richardson Mountains within the Gwich'in people's territory, he said:

> The cold, which seemed to intensify daily or even hourly, appeared to preclude strong winds. Such at least is Kutchin belief. The cold passed the point where experienced and hardened hunters remarked upon it, passed the point where the wood of ax handles and toboggans shattered under stress into chips like glass, and reached the stage where frost appeared to be nipping one's eye balls as well as the usual points: the extremities, ears, nose and cheekbones. Most of us noted difficulty with vision after being outside for a few minutes. This coupled with the widely documented difficulties in judging size and space relationships in the Arctic above timberline, was an added factor in rendering travel impractical for several days. For two days the party camped in a relatively sheltered location. It was during one of these days that a minimum temperature of eighty-three degrees below zero Fahrenheit (minus 63 C) was recorded at Snag, Yukon, some distance to the south.[5]

One very cold January day in Fort McPherson we heard that the temperature had gone down to minus seventy-five degrees (C), and being like the mad dogs and Englishmen who go out in the midday sun, I went out to experience this unique cold spell. Not surprisingly I didn't see anyone else out walking and as the cold bit into me I soon returned to the relative warmth of the nursing station. I had taken off my glasses and put them into my pocket because I knew the frames would get so cold that they would burn the skin on my nose and ears. Now as I entered the station they frosted up even though I had taken them out of my shirt pocket. Contact lenses were in their infancy at that time and the only person who had tried a pair of hard contacts was Alex Forman, the free trader, and his eyes always seemed to look a bit sore. I found wearing glasses a real handicap in the winter, when my glasses would steam up in the warm houses I visited and I had to read a thermometer.

As our oil furnace was having a tough time and seemed to be labouring much more than usual, I went to check our oil supply, which was stored in a large tank inside the utility room. I discovered that the oil was so cold that it had congealed, and in the short distance that it had to go to reach the furnace it did not thaw enough for it to be pumped into the burner. I checked on a barrel of oil outside and it refused to run out of the bung hole when I tipped it over. There was not much we could do except open the oven door and turn up the burner as high as it would go, then put sweaters on and wear our mukluks. Fortunately, this sort of extreme weather only lasted for four or five days, and when the temperature went up to minus thirty (C) it felt positively balmy. But life had to go on, weather or not!

Dave started off slowly, and when the rope was taut, I leaned back and away he went. I immediately fell over into the snow. It took a few trial runs before I had my balance adjusted to the speed of the snowmobile and the drag of the skis in the sugary snow. I discovered that if I leaned too far back, the snowmobile would just spin on the dry snow and ice, but eventually we got everything right and I zoomed over the snow in great style. After about twenty minutes of this, my arms and back ached and I was covered in frost. My face was freezing and my toes were cold, but it had been fun. However, I decided I had had enough and bent down to pick up the skis. To my surprise they were now only about fifteen centimetres wide! The abrasive ice crystals had sanded almost seven centimetres off the soft wood. If I had continued playing around, I would have worn them right out. My curiosity had been satisfied and I never did try it again—even though it was a forerunner to snowboarding!

Both Muriel and I were eager to try all sorts of things out that we had never had an opportunity to do before. We went square dancing, we went curling, we tried cross-country skiing, we drove a dog team and played at being trappers, we built a cabin and went hunting beaver and muskrat in the middle of the night, and whenever the opportunity arose, we tried some jigging, the Gwich'in's traditional dance form. Perhaps the local people thought these young nurses were a bit different, but they all seemed to encourage us to get out there and try these things.

Another challenge came after RCMP Corporal Jim Hickling bought two Honda dirt bikes—small, low-geared automatics painted a beautiful Honda red—and then found himself suddenly transferred to the Eastern Arctic. When he asked us if we were interested in buying the bikes from him, he didn't have to ask twice. Muriel and I soon learned to ride them and used them to do our home visits, strapping a medical bag on the pannier at the back. However, as winter came on, the bikes became stiffer and stiffer in the cold and finally we put them away. Then one very warm spring day when the ice was still strong and the dog team trails were hard-packed, I took one of the bikes out for a test drive. As it hummed along nicely, I went down to the river and followed a trail that had seen heavy loads pulled over it all winter and seemed rock hard. I sped south, delighted how well the bike stayed on the trail. Without any real plan in mind I started to go up the portage leading to Stoney Creek when without warning I found myself standing in creek water by the side of the bike. It happened so quickly I wasn't even sure how it happened! The water had soaked through my mukluks, duffle socks and a pair of thick woolen socks, and as the engine was racing, I knew there was ice stuck in some part of the carburetor. But it was too cold to mess with it, and instead I hauled the bike back onto the trail, turned around and headed for home as quickly as possible. Even though the sun was shining and the day was warm, the temperature was still below freezing, and I could soon feel my mukluks icing up, so as I stood on the bike pedals, it felt as though I was wearing wooden clogs. When I reached the nursing station, I banged up the stairs in my now solid footwear and called to Muriel for help in getting them off.

"The ties are frozen under a pile of ice!" she exclaimed. "What were you thinking of? You'll have to stand in the bathtub to thaw them out."

I clumped over to the bathroom and stood in the tub while she turned on the hot tap. Fortunately my feet did not feel cold and I wasn't worried about them being frozen, but I know they would have been if I had been out much longer. It took several minutes for the ice to begin melting and by then Muriel was laughing at me. "I should take a picture of this—you standing there in your parka and mukluks and taking a bath!"

I laughed, too, but with great relief when Muriel was eventually able to pry off my wet footwear.

But there was one occasion in the early winter when the Honda saved my life or at least saved me from severe injuries. I was driving my bike to the village when a dog team came around a corner and headed toward me. I thought that the noise of the engine would keep them away, but to my consternation and that of the young dog team driver, as soon as the dogs were opposite me, they lunged. I jumped off the bike on the opposite side to them and half-threw the bike toward them. Fortunately, their harnesses got all tangled up in the Honda and I was able to get out of the way and onto the side-walk while the dog musher untangled the harnesses from the bike. I waited until he and his dogs had gone and then retrieved my bike, which was unhurt.

I counted myself very lucky because it was not too long before this episode that the superintendent of the Power Corporation, a man in his mid-fifties, had been walking down the road when a team of dogs went for him. Although he was carrying a big stick and was able to beat them off with the help of the driver, he did suffer bites to his lower legs. Some Mackenzie dogs were ready to attack anything and everything so we were very wary whenever we took our children outdoors, and years later after we moved south they were still scared of strange dogs, even when we met a tiny citi-fied poodle on a leash.

❄ ❄ ❄

In the late 1940s sports were common amongst the Gwich'in people and foot races, canoe races and football (soccer) games were fol-lowed by feasting and dancing. Then, for some unknown reason, af-ter World War Two some sports were curtailed. The anthropologist Richard Slobodin, who spent a number of years among the Gwich'in, was told by the older men that "the young men are too busy drinking homebrew, playing poker, and going into the bushes with the girls to bother with other sports." I'm not sure that much had changed by the sixties, but by then the young people were finding some time for broomball, ice skating and on special occasions like New Year's Day and Easter they would participate in dog team races and snowshoe races. Corporal Bernie Braun, a very popular officer, was instrumen-tal in getting young people involved in sports at that time. Unfortu-nately, when his talents were recognized by his superior officers, he was transferred to Frobisher Bay where youngsters were reportedly causing havoc. Their gain was our loss.

On special occasions there were traditional games for the men and tea-boiling and bannock-making contests for the women, who all looked embarrassed and broke into giggles as crowds gathered around them. Their contests were all done outside where the wood had to be split, a fire made and snow collected and melted before the cooking could begin. In some communities there were rat skinning competitions as well, and though I never watched one, I was told that Mary Firth was the fastest in Fort McPherson, skinning her rat in about thirty seconds. Of course, she had skinned thousands in her lifetime.

In the days when football was played and probably refereed by one of the Scottish Hudson's Bay boys, the field used was the commons area close by the Bay store. The rough ground covered in tufts of grass was matched by an irregularly shaped football made out of a bladder stuffed with moose hair. Sometimes when Eskimo parties had paddled up the Mackenzie and the Peel rivers to trade at the Bay, there would be a football match between the Eskimo and the Gwich'in, which, we were told by Gwich'in men, they always won because the Eskimo men couldn't run as they were too fat! According to Slobodin neither party was better than the other, and success seemed to depend on the element of surprise as much as anything.

Tommy Thrasher was the only Eskimo person living in Fort McPherson, and he was married to a Gwich'in woman named Lucy. Tommy was a muscular man who worked at various jobs in the community, especially where stamina was required, but he also cut firewood, hunted and trapped like the Gwich'in people. However, during the summer months he must have heard the call from his ancestors because he would pack his wife and children into a scow and head off down the Peel and the Mackenzie to the coast where he joined his Eskimo peers on whale hunts. One year after Tommy had been away for several weeks, he reappeared in the settlement and came to ask if I would like to buy some barrels of *muktuk* from him. I had often wondered what *muktuk*, or preserved whale meat, was like after reading that it was an important part of the Eskimo diet. It had been described as having a consistency similar to that of hard-boiled egg white and tasting like the white of an egg, neither of which sounded very appealing to my taste buds.

"Barrels?" I asked incredulously.

"Sure. Your dogs will love it. It'll make their coats nice and shiny and will be good for them in the winter."

It sounded logical because I already fed my dogs with beef fat and fish. What would the difference be? I bought two barrels from him and later in the day Tommy staggered up the hill from his house with a forty-five-gallon barrel balanced precariously in a rickety old wheel barrow.

"Where do you want to keep this? I'll go and get the other one."

I thought I had purchased small ten-gallon barrels of *muktuk*, but now I could see that this would last my dogs throughout the whole winter. "Put them in the warehouse, please," I said. "It's warm in there and will be handy to mix with the other dog feed."

One day after the cold weather came later in the year as I was preparing some dog feed, I opened the top of one of the barrels. I was not expecting the smell and had to rush out into the fresh air. Then carefully re-entering with a cloth over my nose and mouth, I peered into the barrel. Large globs of a white, leathery-looking substance were floating on top of a greasy, oily liquid. I wondered if it would kill my dogs if I fed it to them, but one way or the other I knew I had to use it or get rid of it. If I tipped it outside of the warehouse, no one would want to come near, so I tentatively scooped some of the mess into a pail and carried it toward the dogs. As I approached, they howled and barked because they recognized the pail as the feeding bucket. I sloshed some down into one of the dog's feeding dishes and waited. He sniffed it suspiciously and then licked it, and finding that it was just fine, he picked up a piece of the muktuk, took two bites of it and then swallowed it. I just about gagged.

I watched him for a few moments and as he didn't keel over, I went back and fed some to the rest of the dogs, holding my breath every time I dipped the bucket into the barrel. Over the next few weeks I started mixing some of it with the cereal that the dogs were usually fed and they did fine. One day William Firth went into the warehouse and came staggering right out again. He asked what on earth I had in there that had gone rotten, so I told him about Tommy's *muktuk*.

"You have to be careful with that stuff from the coast, you know," he said. "Some of the people have died from eating old seal flippers. They get botulism."

"William, there is no way I am going to eat any of that stuff out there! It's only for the dogs."

"Well, you be careful!" He was very distrustful of anything from the coast, and yet in his earlier years he had travelled quite extensively by dog team in that area.

I was very careful and wore gloves and an old coat whenever I served any of the *muktuk* up to my dogs, but not because I was worried about botulism. I was only concerned that, if I got some of it on me, I wouldn't be able to get rid of the smell and I would be having a very lonely winter!

One New Year's Day it was announced that there would be dog team races starting at the creek over the river, crossing the river and going up the road that led into the village. Because the dogs were vicious and would fight any other dog or team that came close, the race was to be a timed event. As I frequently took my dog team across the river and up the small creek where we had our small cabin, they were familiar with this route, although I'd had some hair-raising trips with them, especially when travelling home in the dark. At the bottom of the hill that went up to the village I would yell, "Cha!" and the dogs would swing to the left and within a few minutes we would arrive at the point below the nursing station where I kept them tied up.

With some trepidation I signed up for the race, and after making the trip a few more times I became confident that we could cross the finishing line in good time. The day of the event came and I had the dogs all harnessed up and ready to go. I was excited and they seemed to sense that this was something special as they stood braced in their harnesses, and now and again one would bark and I noticed that my leader was shaking with the anticipation.

When it was my turn and the racer before me had gone up the hill, I unfastened my sled, took my foot off the brake that was dug deep into the snow and we set off across the river. The dogs just flew along with the empty, flat-bottomed oak toboggan bouncing over the wind drifts on the snow. Off the river and over the sand bar then over the narrow log bridge we went, and we were just ready to go up the hill to the finishing line when my leader swerved so sharply and unexpectedly to the left, taking the rest of the team with him, that I was thrown off the toboggan and landed in a snow drift.

"You stupid, stupid dog!" I yelled. "Just wait until I catch you, you miserable hound!"

I could have saved my breath. I brushed the snow off my parka and walked down the trail in disgust, embarrassed that I had fallen off in front of the crowd of onlookers and that my dogs had been stupid enough to want to go home. When I reached the dogs, they were snarling at each other because each one was trying to lie down by his own box and the harness was restricting them. I quickly unharnessed them before a fight could start and chained them to their posts. I was still so mad that I didn't even pet them as I usually did.

I met Muriel after I had heaved myself up the snowy bank. "That didn't work out at all well," I said breathlessly. "In fact, it was a real shmozzle."

"You looked as though you were making a really fast trip when I saw you, then you just seemed to disappear!"

"I guess my dogs just like home so much that all they think about is bed and food."

"Like someone else I know!" Muriel said with a laugh.

I had to laugh. "That reminds me, it must be coffee time and I know you made cinnamon rolls. I'll feed the dogs later."

We went inside and I took my frustration out on the still warm cinnamon rolls.

There is nothing like a dog team for getting you where you want to go in the North—if you are not racing, that is—and with dogs there are no problems associated with the energy crisis and no long-lasting pollution. But driving a working dog team may bring out some of the things in a person's character that should be left dormant, and I have been exasperated many times and amused just as many times by my dogs' behaviour. Several times I was reduced to laughter over an incident that had at first made me boiling mad. For instance, many a time when I was leaving the village with my dogs, all of them fresh and eager to go, and hurtling down the riverbank, the toboggan skipping over the frozen ice, one of the dogs toward the front would decide that he had to stop and relieve himself. It seemed that this always happened just as I was glancing behind me, and it would result in absolute chaos as the toboggan ploughed into the dogs who had all stopped, and I was thrown over the lazyback into the carriole. And I had to learn to avoid words such as "Oh no!" or "So?" when in general conversation with someone riding in the carriole because the dogs would immediately stop, thinking they heard something that sounded like "Whoa!" which is what they really wanted to hear.

The dogs in my team had distinct personalities. My leader, Silver, was a silver and grey dog from Siberian stock, but he probably had inherited some genes from a stray Mackenzie River husky because he would fight other dogs without too much provocation. As the leader, he may have had to maintain his dominance in the pack, but I could trust him around our children and he acted like a little puppy with them. Like all the dogs, Silver was chained to a post close to the property fence, and although he had a box to shelter in if he wanted to, he had the most peculiar habit of balancing himself on top of the chain-link fence, which was folded over at the top, and from there he would look down on the other dogs with an air of superiority. Muriel said she thought that he must have been crossed with a rooster!

Ginger was a dog of that colour who kept to himself, rarely fought and was probably a bit simple. His large ears stuck out at right angles and the only time he got excited was at feeding time. When he was young, I tried him in the lead position as I had tried each of the dogs, looking for one that had the greatest potential in that post, and as long as the trail went straight ahead, Ginger worked well. However, if we came to a cross-trail, even something as insignificant as a mouse trail, he would immediately turn off to follow it.

The two beautiful pups I was given by the RCMP in Arctic Red River became good sled dogs. I had been at a loss what to call them and came up with the name Thursday for one because that was the day on which I obtained them, and because you can't have two dogs named Thursday the other one became Friday.

Adaijoh was my wheel dog—the one who runs next to the toboggan. I gave him that name because he was big and hairy and I had heard it was the nickname that some of the Gwich'in had given to me as it meant "whiskers!" Adaijoh was as bright as his brother, Silver, and between them they kept the toboggan on track. He would lean to the right when we were turning left so the toboggan would stay on the trail and not get pulled off by the rest of the team. He could fight but only got involved in self-defence.

A tall, fairly skinny Siberian dog came to me from Old Crow where he had been a member of the RCMP dog team patrol. He had incurred the wrath of the Mounties during their last patrol from Old Crow to Fort McPherson because, when they were going down hills, he had braked instead of pulling and had torn his footpads badly. I think he may have been rear-ended by a toboggan too many times when he was a pup with the result that he had become a little timid going down hills at speed. Thinking that he would be of no further use, they gave him to me after he was officially "put down." As it was Easter weekend when he arrived, that is what I named him. I kept him tied up for a few weeks, gave him penicillin in his feed, and when his footpads looked as though they had healed, I put him in harness. When we came to a hill, I rode the brake and shouted encouragement to him (and the others, of course) and he soon learned to pull downhill. He turned out to be an excellent dog.

(I was not very good at giving my dogs real northern names like "Chimo" or even "King" as in the radio series "Sergeant Preston of the Mounties," which had featured Preston calling "On, King, on, you husky!" When I was calling my dogs, it sounded like I was looking forward to a weekend holiday—"C'mon, Thursday, Friday and Easter!")

When I first learned that the northern sled dog's diet was mostly fish, I was quite surprised as I thought only cats ate fish. The fish the dogs ate on the trail had sometimes been dried and smoked to preserve it but it was used because it was light to carry on long trips. At home they were fed fresh or frozen fish that they quickly devoured. On the last trip I made to Arctic Red River late one spring, I took a young social worker from Inuvik on a one-way trip with me. At our destination Special Constable Joe Masazumi fed my dogs pit fish, a horrible mess of half-rotten fish that had been lying all winter in a pit dug into the permafrost. A few hours later as we were travelling back in the hot sun, the dogs started throwing up, and I was surprised to see whole fish skeletons regurgitated and wondered how the dogs had even managed to swallow them without chewing. I was glad that the young social worker was not with me to photograph this unflattering side of dog team travel.

When the dogs were working well and the snow conditions were good for travelling, I could feel a real high at the sheer exhilaration of racing across the glistening snow, being pulled by eager, happy dogs. I would talk to the dogs sometimes just to remind them that I was still there, and when we went swooping down a hill, I would give a shrill "Wheee!" which seemed to infect them with the same enthusiasm. But during the day they would sometimes lose their enthusiasm and I would crack my whip to remind them that they were working dogs. By the end of the day they would be pulling like automatons with no stops, not even to pee, as if they knew the days' work was nearly over.

Summer was a tough time for all the sled dogs in the North, and it is a wonder that many of them survived. In the old days as soon as the snows melted and the dogs were not needed, they were turned loose, and although they had easy access to water, they ate whatever they could find or steal. When it became mandatory to fasten up the dogs in a village, they were often lucky to get food every few days. Water, which had to be carried from the river, was quite scarce. They would be given a bucket of fresh water and, dogs being dogs, would almost immediately knock it over as they ran in circles around the pole to which they were chained. There were always one or two that would break their chains and run around the village, and the dogs that were still tied up would lunge at these strays and quite often break their chains, and then there would be a horrendous dogfight. My dogs were quite fortunate in being tied up on the nursing station grounds because water and food were quite easily accessible, and if I was away, William Firth would feed them for me. Later after William had retired, Albert Peterson took over from him and was equally as helpful. But after they had been tied up all summer, when they were put into harness in the fall, I found that it took them about three good runs before their stamina returned.

In the early spring of 1969 the opportunity came for Muriel and I and our two children to spend a few days camping, after Phyllis Seaton, the wife of the Hudson's Bay manager, offered to take care of the nursing station if we wanted a few days away. Phyllis was a nurse with nursing-station experience and we felt very fortunate and thankful that we could take a break with our family and not have to worry about any emergencies. We decided we would take our dog team up Stoney Creek and camp in a sheltered location for a few days to do some local exploring. A few years earlier we had winter-camped at the head of this creek for a few days and been caught in a severe Arctic windstorm, sometimes called a williwaw, and seen

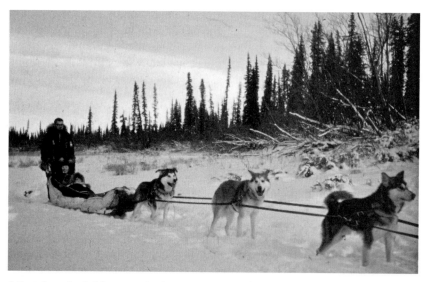

Muriel and children tucked into the family bus, with three of five dogs showing.

and felt small stones and sharp shale being blown horizontally down the creek. During the night a large spruce tree next to our tent had blown over, scaring us and the children. But now the weather was just comfortably cold, around the minus thirty mark, and there was no sign of storms on the horizon.

We gathered our food, dog food, tent and stove, caribou skins for sleeping on and all the other paraphernalia that goes along with winter camping, and I packed the toboggan carefully, making sure that there was some room for Muriel and the two children and a few toys. Waving to Phyllis and then to William Firth, who had come to check that we had everything—"Don't forget matches, and keep your axe handy!"—I drove the dogs down onto the Peel River and headed south toward the mouth of Stoney Creek. There was a good trail with hard-packed snow because caribou hunters had been travelling to and from the mountains hauling meat, so we were able to make good time, and the dogs, their tails held high, seemed to enjoy their work even though the toboggan was very heavily loaded.

The sun shone down on us out of a deep blue sky and the snow

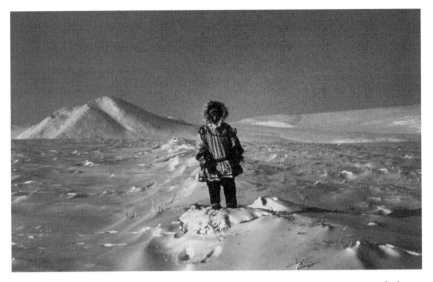

Helen took everything in her stride as if this was the most natural thing in the world.

sparkled in the sunlight. The spruce trees that lined the river looked intensely green against the blue sky and the dazzling white snow, and our spirits soared as we left twenty-four-hour-a-day responsibilities behind at the nursing station. Muriel especially appreciated being away from the daily grind and out in the open spaces as she rarely got to visit the mountain camps, not wanting to travel alone or with a group of men as I did.

As we went up Stoney Creek, the rocky bluffs on either side of the creek got higher and higher, and above us huge black ravens floated effortlessly on the wind currents, calling to each other with their raucous croaking. Some of them, sitting on the high rocks, made unique hollow sounds like empty pipes being struck with a hammer, and once again I thought it was not surprising that there were so many superstitions about these birds.

We stopped periodically to rest the dogs and to let Muriel and the children stretch their legs, but as we carried a Thermos of hot chocolate with us, I didn't have to light a fire and everyone was quite warm without one. Later when we stopped for lunch, I made a big

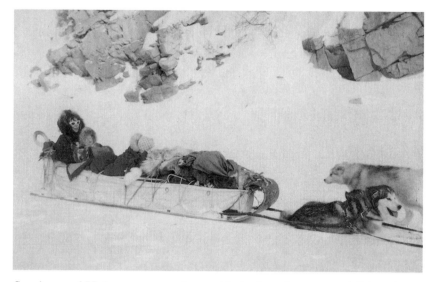

Stephen and Helen, as snug as bugs, ride in the toboggan with Muriel.

fire and cut some spruce branches to put around it for us to sit on, and it was very much a picnic, which Helen and Stephen decided was a lot of fun. The dogs buried their faces in the snow and took large gulps of it to slake their thirst then lay in the sun panting and watching us.

By mid-afternoon we had travelled almost to the head of the creek and I stopped the team at a point that was sheltered from the wind and where there was enough wood for a fire and green brush for the floor of the tent. After I had tied up the dogs and given them brush to lie on, we unloaded the toboggan and let the children play in it while Muriel and I set our canvas tent up. Then Muriel laid brush on the floor of the tent while I cut firewood, using a large bow saw.

By this time the sun was getting low and we began to notice the cold, but the stove was soon up and running with thick smoke pouring from its chimney and its heat was soon quite noticeable inside the tent.

After supper, the children played on the caribou skins that we had laid down over the green boughs, and though we didn't think about it until later, they took everything in their stride as if camping was the most natural thing in the world. At bedtime, we dressed them in bunny suits—pajamas with long sleeves and pant legs with attached bootees—so if the covers came off them during the night they would not get too cold. Muriel read them a story by the light of our Coleman gas lamp and they soon drifted off to sleep. Muriel and I caught up on our own reading, and then after I had filled the stove and made some firesticks for the morning, we crawled into our sleeping bags to listen to CHAK's "Neighbourly News and Messages" on our portable radio.

It was very relaxing, lying there in the dark listening to the fire crackling and spitting, smelling the sweet smell of the green boughs beneath us and breathing the rapidly cooling air.

Then suddenly Muriel sat up. "I can smell burning plastic!" I leapt out of my sleeping bag, grabbed a flashlight and saw that the radio had slipped down beside the stove. One side of the radio had melted and the control for changing the station was adhered to the case, but when I turned it on and heard CHAK quite clearly, I breathed a sigh of relief. There were no other stations to tune in to so I wasn't bothered about having it set forever on CHAK.

Sometime during the night I awoke as the dogs had all started howling in unison, possibly singing to some unseen relatives. Then as suddenly as a tap being turned off, they abruptly stopped, and I found that I was listening intently, for what? A reply? I smiled, turned over, found my dislodged toque, pulled it down over my ears and went back to sleep.

After breakfast the next morning I cut and split some more wood before we harnessed up the dogs and went farther up the creek. Then with Muriel handling the toboggan with the children in it, I put on my snowshoes and made a trail out of the creek and up onto the tundra. There we stopped and ate the sandwiches that Muriel had made and shared the Thermos of hot chocolate. As we were eating, we saw two dog teams in the distance coming toward us. I didn't recognize either of them and I was pretty sure there were no hunters in this area, but as they came closer, I could see that the dogs in one team were all Siberian Huskies, which only the RCMP used.

When the teams reached us, they stopped and we were surprised to learn that they were Mounties from Old Crow. Peter Benjamin was a Gwich'in special constable, and he was the guide for Constable Warren Townsend on what was to be the last RCMP dog team patrol from Old Crow to Fort McPherson and Arctic Red River and then back again—a round-trip of almost a thousand kilometres. They had been held up on the other side of the mountains for two days by very high winds and blizzards and now they were looking forward to getting to Fort McPherson. We were the first people they had met as they neared their destination, and afterwards when I thought about this historic patrol, I realized that it must have been a bit of a letdown when the first people they met at the top of that last mountain pass were a couple of white English nurses and their two tiny children! I told them where our tent was set and invited them to go in, make tea and get warm as the stove probably still had wood burning in it. They followed our trail down the mountain to our camp, and by the time we returned to it several hours later, they had been and gone.

We spent one more night in the camp, then the next morning after breakfast we packed everything up, pulled down the tent and headed for home. The weather had stayed sunny and we were sorry that we couldn't stay out longer, but we did not want to presume too much on Phyllis's kindness. We arrived home to a quiet nursing station and soon the children were playing in their bedroom as though they had never been away, except that both of them had very red faces from the cold and the sun.

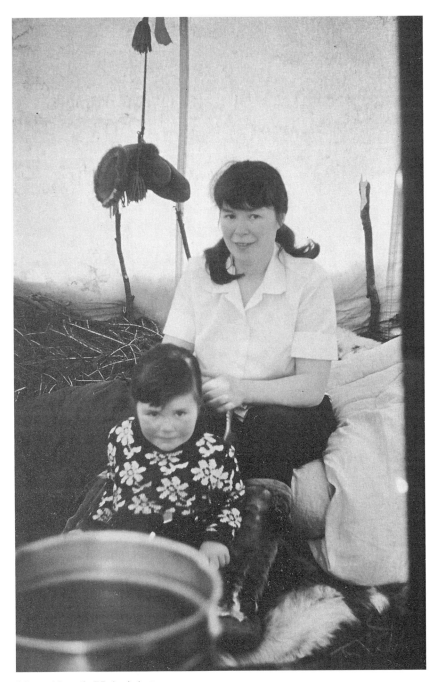

Muriel braids Helen's hair at camp.

CHAPTER TWELVE

ARLY SPRING BEFORE BREAKUP WAS A busy time in the village, with people coming and going either to their hunting camps in the mountains or to their muskrat camps in the Delta. Mary Firth did not have far to go to her trapline as it was just across the river, but she told us she only played at trapping and her earnings just provided her with pocket money. Like every trapline, hers was registered in her name and no one else could trap on it without her permission, but sometimes she would take Muriel and me over and show us how to set the traps, and she would laugh out loud when I tried to set the spring and it would go off and make me jump back nervously. When we went back with her a day or two later, she was always very excited when she had caught something.

Since muskrats are weed feeders, they harvest bunches of grassy weeds from the bottom of the lake and bring them to the surface where they eat some and use the rest to build their small shelters on the surface of the ice so their access holes stay unfrozen. In the late spring when the snow had melted and settled, the muskrat houses can be plainly seen, when there is no more fresh snow to cover them. However, during the winter these houses are covered by snow, although Mary could identify them by the small mound that showed under the drifts. After clearing the snow away with her arm, she would open one side of a grassy mound with her axe and then set her small trap on the little icy platform that the muskrat used when

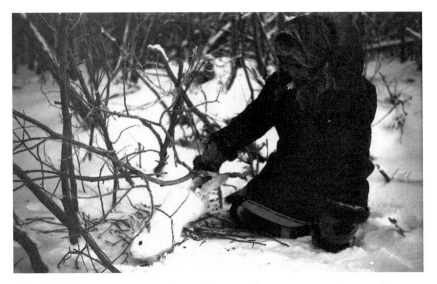

Mary Firth inspects a snowshoe rabbit caught in a snare at her trapline.

it sat there to eat. The trap was held in place by a thin chain attached to a piece of wood. The idea was, Mary explained, that the muskrat would swim up to the hole in the ice and heave itself out and presto! he would get his foot caught in the trap. When she reopened the house a day or two later one of three things could have occurred: the rat would be alive and sitting on his platform with his foot in the trap, the rat had drowned when the trap was sprung and he fell back into the water or the trap would be full of brown soggy weeds.

After returning home with her catch of the day, she would fasten the rat's hind legs to a chair back and with a sharp knife, take the skin off without inflicting a single cut in it. Then she would put each skin onto a stretcher board with the fur side in, put in a few tacks to hold it in place and hang it up in the house to dry. Next she would clean the muskrat carcasses, the offal going into the dogs' pot to be fed to them later, and the meat washed and put into a baking pan where it looked to me like the chicken thighs sold in the meat departments of southern grocery stores. I didn't taste any, although Mary said that when it was baked or roasted, it tasted like fatty chicken. The rat tails were not wasted, either. They were dipped into

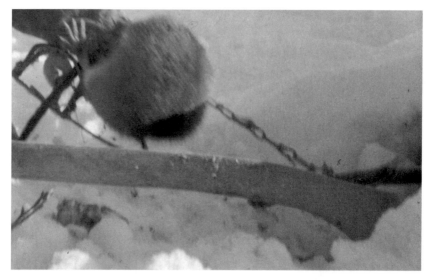

Muskrat trapping was the livelihood that Gwich'in people relied on.

boiling water to remove the hair and then roasted. Of course, these rats are quite different from the southern vermin rat (*Rattus rattus*). Muskrats (*Ondatra zibethicus*) are like miniature beaver with partially webbed feet. Their common name comes from their mild, unobjectionable musty odour that Mary said does not affect the taste of the meat, and as they are very clean animals, they would make quite a satisfactory diet—for those who don't have anything else!

Periodically Muriel and I would cross the Peel River and walk Mary's trapline because it was a place we could go by ourselves on snowshoes and feel as though we were far out in the bush, getting a taste of what everyday life was like for the trappers. Mary did not set many traps, so if we had some extra time, we would take over our dog team and go from lake to lake to check them. After we had visited them a few times, our dogs became accustomed to the routine and came to know where the traps were located. When a heavy snowfall had obliterated all signs of the houses, my lead dog would still go unerringly from trap to trap and then stop without me saying a word to him. When he stopped, I knew there must be a trap in the vicinity, and I would feel around in the snow with my foot until

180

I located the hard lump that indicated the muskrat house.

One day it seemed as though the dogs were on "automatic" because they stopped at each rat house on their own, and when I had checked it, covered it with snow again and thrown the axe into the sled, they would move off for the next rat house without waiting for a command. This worked fine until the dogs decided to move just as Muriel was bending over to get into the sled. The carriole's lazyback struck her backside and knocked her headfirst into the deep snow. It was hilarious to see her legs kicking in the snow, but when I went over to help her get up, she hadn't found it at all funny because she couldn't breathe and was being asphyxiated. By the time we caught up to the dogs at the next rat house, she had begun to see the funny side of it, although I could now see how dangerous being buried in snow could be.

One of Mary's boys caught a good-sized beaver and she asked if we would like to see how it was prepared. This beaver weighed about sixty-five kilos and she skinned it on the floor because it was too heavy to hold up any other way. When she was finished, she laid the skin out flat with the fur down, nailing it to a large plywood board where it would stay for several days until it was dry. Then she cleaned the large, flat beaver tail and roasted it by an open fire; I tried it but it was chewy and fatty and did not suit my taste at all.

Beaver traps were set on the rivers or lakes as soon as the ice was strong enough to bear a man's weight, but the job was labour intensive. A pole with a little platform attached to it was prepared and then the trap was placed on the platform and wired to the pole. After a hole had been chopped in the ice, the pole was thrust down to the bottom of the lake or river. Whenever the trap was checked, the ice had once again to be chopped open and the pole and possibly a heavy beaver had to be heaved to the surface and removed and the trap re-set. The beaver was then hauled back to the cabin or tent where it was skinned and the pelt fastened to either a large hoop or nailed onto a board. But beaver would also take advantage of the spring sun and come out to bask like lazy seals, and when located, the holes from which they emerged could be utilized for setting a trap. The game warden gave out discs that had to be fastened to the beaver pelts before they were shipped out or traded at the Bay, so no one minded when Muriel and I went to Mary's trapline and caught something because they knew we couldn't sell it without the necessary legal tag, and we always gave everything to Mary anyway.

Some people were very good at trapping and took care of the furs, but others were not as industrious and didn't check their traps regularly so there was a greater risk of the fur being damaged in the trap or by some other animal. Mary told us that the fur that was not good enough to sell was home-tanned and used for trimming moccasins, gloves or parkas or making doll clothes, but it was never wasted.

It seems cruel to many people, but one trapper told us that if these animals weren't trapped they would soon be dying of hunger because there would not be enough food for them all or they would get diseases because of overcrowding and fighting. "People who complain about trapping wear leather shoes and eat beef and bacon. Where do they suppose that comes from?" was a sentiment I heard from different sources over the years. Most trappers looked upon their occupation as a farmer would, rotating their traps as a farmer rotates his fields and crops.

There are, of course, some unpleasant aspects to trapping, as we found out on one of our early forays along Mary's trapline when we found a mink that was still alive in a trap. I had carried my .22 along with me in case we saw a rabbit or two, so I thought I would dispatch the mink with a .22 short. Fortunately, as it turned out, snow had got into the breech of my unprotected rifle, and the bolt would only cruise down slowly to the shell without firing it. After a few tries I gave up and, not knowing how else to kill the mink, we returned and told Mary about it. She was very excited and immediately got ready to visit the trap. "That mink, he's worth lots of money at this time of the year. Lucky you didn't shoot it. You could have spoiled the fur!" I asked her how she would kill it, and when she told me she would stab it in the mouth with a stick, I knew I wouldn't have been able to do that.

On another visit to Mary's traps, Muriel and I also snowshoed over to check the rabbit snares she had set. When we arrived, we saw something in the bushes that looked too large for a rabbit so we approached it carefully and were surprised to see a great horned owl had been caught in the snare. It glared at us and made hissing noises and backed away to the limit of the snare wire.

How it had got in there was a mystery to us because the snare had been set in a tangle of willows and I thought that owls, like other predatory birds, swooped down on their unsuspecting prey and carried them off. But perhaps this owl had been in pursuit of a rabbit, although it could not have been flying in this thick undergrowth and I don't think an owl could walk very fast!

I had thick gloves on and tried approaching it, but it seemed to get bigger and bigger the closer I got, and it was certainly not welcoming my advance. I have to admit that I was a bit timid at handling this rather aggressive bird, which raised its wings so that it looked much bigger, and as it held this threatening posture it hissed at us while fixing us with its impressive large staring eyes. As usual, when confronted with an unknown on Mary's trapline, we went back to tell her, but she had never experienced anything like this before, so she sent one of her adult children over to investigate. He returned later with the dead bird; it had been impossible for him to release it and he had to kill it as it would have eventually died in the snare. He took the bird to the school where he thought one of the teachers would help the children to skin, preserve and mount the owl as an educational tool.

Rabbits have a seven-year population cycle and we assumed that they must be at their peak when Mary Firth set a dozen or so snares on her trapline. "What do you do with all the skins, Mary?" I asked when she came back carrying a bag full of rabbits and called at the nursing station to see if we wanted one for supper.

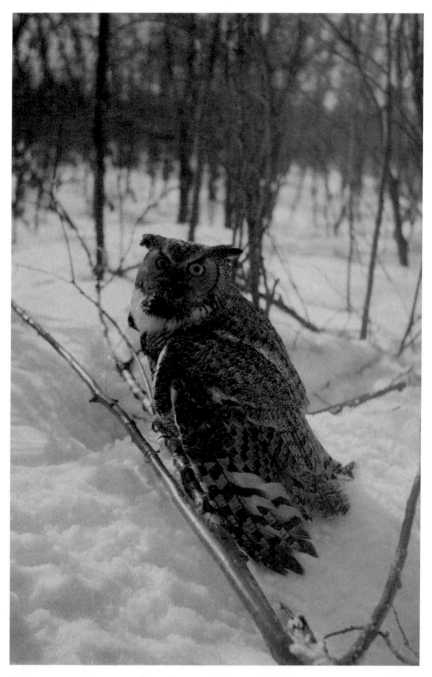

It was a mystery to us how this great horned owl became entrapped in a rabbit snare.

"Can you sell them?"

"No, no one wants them now. I just chuck them or let the dogs have them."

William, who was taking an afternoon break, spoke up. "In the old days they were used for making blankets and baby clothes and they were worn inside mukluks before duffle socks were used."

"Does anyone still remember how to make them?" Muriel asked, looking into the bag of rabbits and then running her fingers over the fur. "I have seen some of the people with rabbit fur on their slippers."

Mary told us that some of the old women in the village probably still knew how to do it, and then William said his mother used to start by drying the skins, then after cutting them in long strips, she would wind them around long pieces of thong made from soft caribou skin until there was enough to hand-weave a garment or a blanket. As Mary went out, she offered to ask around and see if someone would make us a rabbit-skin coat for our daughter, Helen, who was nearly one year old.

A month later Mary knocked quietly on the back door, and when we opened it, we saw that Elizabeth Kunnizzi was with her and Elizabeth was carrying a paper-wrapped parcel. Elizabeth did not speak very much English, preferring to speak her own language, and she had brought Mary with her to translate.

"Elizabeth, she's got something for you," Mary said. "It's really nice!"

They came in and Muriel put the kettle on for tea, then as we sat around the kitchen table, Elizabeth pushed the parcel toward Muriel. "Open it," she instructed. Muriel opened the parcel to reveal a small rabbit-skin parka, which looked as though it would just fit Helen. We fetched our daughter from the playroom and tried it on her. The parka was hooded and the long sleeves were closed at the end like having sewn-on gloves, a valuable addition for small children out in the cold. Helen sat on the carpet and smiled up at us. She seemed to like it, too, and I think the rabbit hair tickled her nose.

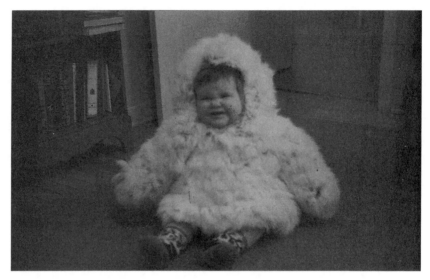

Helen wears a ticklish snowshoe rabbit parka.

We asked Elizabeth how much she wanted for it but she just smiled and looked at Mary. They talked back and forth in Gwich'in for a few minutes.

"Well?" Muriel asked.

"She said give her whatever you think." Very few of the women would come right out and give a price for their work.

Muriel made an offer and after the women had conferred, Mary said exactly what we had expected her to say. "That's too much. The coat, it's not very good."

Muriel insisted on giving a cheque to Elizabeth who took it even as she was saying, "No, no, too much. Massi cho!"

We hoped it was enough because it was not very much to us when we considered the work that had gone into the project, but Mary assured us that Elizabeth was quite happy with the money. Later when William came around, we showed the little parka to him and he explained that the women "sort of knit them with their fingers. They don't use knitting needles." And he intertwined his fingers to demonstrate. "It's like making a fishnet but without the shuttle."

We examined the parka and saw that it was constructed with

large mesh openings, which the rabbit fur filled, and thus the hair and the air pockets provided excellent insulation. When Helen woke up from an afternoon nap we tried the parka on her again and it really did fit beautifully, but it was a challenge to pull her arms through the sleeves without getting her fingers caught in the mesh.

I told William I was going to have a go at making a blanket if I could get hold of enough skins and he promised to ask Mary to keep all the ones she got. As rabbit skins were brought in, not only by Mary but by some of her friends, too, I hung them in our warehouse to dry. Then one weekend when I had what seemed like countless dozens of them, I started cutting them into strips. Instead of moose-hide thongs or babiche, I twisted the strips of fur around some sisal string, and before long it stretched from one end of the warehouse to the other and back again. Then William came to show me how he thought that I should tie or knit it, and over the next few days I made a narrow blanket that was about one metre by two, enough to go over Helen when we took her out in her little sled. It was warm but we found that afterwards we and everything we touched were covered in rabbit hair. However, I asked myself if this would have mattered if we had lived in a tent in the old days.

Maybe because of the profession I was in, I found that killing anything was very difficult and somewhat abhorrent. Once when I was at a caribou hunting camp and the young men had shot some caribou, one of the animals had been severely wounded in the legs and couldn't walk. It was close to the camp and old Jim Vittrekwa told me to go and get it. "But I don't have a gun!" I told him. "Well, use your knife," and he indicated the long sheath knife I had at my belt. Not wanting to appear stupid in front of this grizzled hunter, I climbed the icy slope to where the caribou was sitting and staring at me with its big doleful eyes.

I pulled out my knife and looked at the caribou. Okay, now what? Jim's brother William had shown me where to stab an animal to kill it quickly and this involved sticking the knife in at the base of the skull. I was facing the animal, and every time I went to move around it, it struggled and kicked with its broken legs but it could not move away. I was as nervous as the caribou and finally I lunged forward and grabbed hold of one its large antlers. I was surprised how strong it was, considering that it had been so wounded, but I managed to get in the right position and held my knife in what I hoped was the correct spot. I shut my eyes tight and pushed the knife with all my strength. Nothing happened. I had hit bone just underneath the skin. Still holding the knife and hanging onto one of the antlers, I felt around with my finger until I hit a depression that I thought should be the right spot and, placing the point of the knife there, I lunged. The caribou went into spasm and I knew I had severed its spinal cord. But its eyes seemed to get bigger as it looked at me with what I felt was reproach, and although I knew that, if left alone, it would have died a prolonged death or been killed by wolves, I felt sad that I had to kill such a beautiful animal. I pushed its head down into a snowbank so it couldn't look at me and held it there until all movement ceased, then I used the belt that held up my pants and pulled the caribou carcass down the mountain to the camp.

"We'll use it for dog feed," Jim said. This was rather an ignominious end for an animal that had travelled hundreds of kilometres across the tundra, and I wondered if the meat would somehow taste a bit different when the animal had not been killed quickly or because I had not gutted it immediately. But the dogs would have been fed with caribou meat one way or another, so I told myself it was good that it would not be wasted.

In April 1968 when muskrat trapping was in full swing, Fort McPherson became very quiet. Most of the people were out at their camps in the Mackenzie Delta and their school-aged children were safely in the school hostel. Even some of the older people, if they were at all mobile, had elected to go with the younger people out to the camps where they could live as close as possible to the traditional Gwich'in life. All of this made me want to visit them in their rat

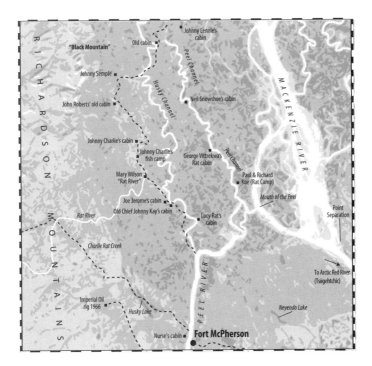

The route around the Delta that Corporal Shane Hennan and I took followed the trail to the rat camps.

camps to see firsthand how they lived, and because whole families were out there, I could check on their health and perhaps offer some healthy advice. Muriel agreed that I should go and we discussed the families that would be out there in the Delta so I was up to date on their various ailments.

I went around to the RCMP office to let them know that I was planning a trip to the Delta within the next few days, and just in case they had to come and rescue me, I pointed out my intended route on the big map pinned to their office wall. Before I could go into the details, Corporal Shane Hennan told me that he had been contemplating a trip himself, but since he had not travelled with dogs in that area before, he was looking for someone to travel with. "If I can get some dogs and a toboggan—if there are any left in town—would you mind some company to the Delta?" This was the second time

189

that this had happened to me, not that I minded, and I facetiously thought of applying for a guide's license!

Travelling with Shane would make the trip more enjoyable, and even if the conditions became really bad, it would be nice to share the misery. The only problem I could envisage was that when some of the people saw a member of the RCMP approaching their cabins, they might become defensive, whereas I had always been welcomed very warmly at all the local camps I visited when I travelled alone or with Muriel. But when I mentioned this concern to Muriel, she told me that she would feel much more comfortable if Shane was with me and admitted that she had been a bit worried at the thought of me going alone. Shane would make a pleasant travelling companion as he was a fairly quiet man—considering he was a Mountie—and I looked forward to his company.

When William Firth came around to the house later that day and I told him that Shane might go with me if he could find some dogs and equipment, William immediately offered to lend his team. "They aren't speedy, but they will get there if the corporal knows how to drive them."

I thought that even if Shane didn't know much about them at first, it wouldn't take long before he did. Having a dog team is like having children—you learn as you go! Shane and I agreed to meet in the morning down on the river after the dogs were over their first excited mad dash, and then we could travel down the trail like civilized dog mushers. I hauled my toboggan into our small warehouse to tighten the babiche fastenings and then piled up my food, the dog food, a winter sleeping bag, an axe and a can of kerosene-soaked rags to be used to make quick fires. I then packed my stethoscope, a blood pressure monitor, a hemaglobinometer and a supply of medicines.

By eight-fifteen the next morning, I was ready to leave. The April weather was beautiful, the sun shining out of a clear blue sky. There was no wind and the temperature was close to minus twenty (C). At my command the dogs tightened the harness and I unfastened the rope that tethered the toboggan to a post. I yelled "Alright!" and the dogs shot out of the yard. The first few minutes were exhilarating as the dogs sped down toward the frozen river with the heavily loaded toboggan gliding smoothly on the hard-packed road. They seemed to sense that I was excited, too, and ran with their tails held high. But my exhilaration was short lived. Coming to the trail leading down to the river, I yelled for the dogs to turn left, and they did it with such gusto that I lost control of the toboggan and did a belly flop into a snow-bank. Fortunately, the toboggan tipped as I fell and careened into a snowbank where it and the dogs were pulled to a stop. As I extricated myself, they lunged into the soft snow, wagging their tails and gulping large mouthfuls of snow. When I ran down and straightened up the toboggan, I saw that a piece of the runner next to the brake had broken off, but fortunately it would not make the toboggan drag. A small part that held the two handles of the lazyback together had also broken in the collision with the hard ice, but it wasn't serious so I quickly straightened out the dogs and continued down the trail. Shane would be showing up on the riverbank any minute and I did not want to get run down by his dog team.

I had only been on the trail again for a few minutes when I glanced back and saw that Shane was about twenty metres behind me. I waved, and seeing all was well, we both travelled north down the river. The dogs ran so well we did not have much opportunity to get off and run behind them, and consequently we were both chilled by the time we arrived at the first cabin. After banging on the door, we gathered that there was no one home. It was unlocked, so we went in and made a fire in the old wood stove. As soon as the cabin was warm and we had thawed out, we ate our lunches and then looked around at the cabin interior. By the look of it, it was not a residence cabin but may have been just used as we were using it, as a place to stop and warm up out of the wind, or perhaps it was only used in the summertime. The log walls were festooned with messages, some written with a felt pen, others in pencil and some with the end of a burned stick. Someone with more time on his hands had cut letters from a cereal box and stuck them on the wall with candle fat to spell out the titles of popular songs, while here and there were the usual graffiti drawings that said with many variations that "Abe loves Mary."

By the time we finished lunch it was well after noon, and having read the walls, we reluctantly put on our parkas and went out to the dogs who were curled up in the snow. We only fed the dogs at the end of the day because the old men who advised us on driving dogs said that they would not work on full stomachs. The only time we did not adhere to this rule was when the temperature plunged to minus thirty or colder, and then we gave them each a half pound of beef fat (locally called tallow) to combat the cold.

One long bushy portage and a short run on the river took us to the Mouth of the Peel where it emptied its muddy waters into the mighty Mackenzie River. In the old days this junction had been in the buffer zone between the Eskimo people of the coast and the Gwich'in of the mountains, but for more than a hundred years people had camped here seasonally, and now there was a small collection of cabins known as "The Mouth of the Peel." An old man came to the door of one of the cabins and invited us in. Jimmy Thompson was an elder from Fort McPherson, and he and his wife spent each spring at this cabin while they were ratting, then after a brief visit to Fort McPherson for supplies, they would come back here for the excellent fishing. Within a few weeks they would be able to put up all the fish they needed for dog feed for the following winter.

Shane and I declined tea, but hearing that Peter Nerysoo had recently passed through heading for Mackenzie Island, we decided to carry on before it got dark. After travelling on Peter's trail for awhile, we turned off and headed west up the branch of the river that went past Aklavik, although we did not intend to travel that far. Expecting that we would now have to break trail, we were delighted to see traces of old tracks from the game warden's Bombardier, a large twin-tracked vehicle powered by a V8 engine. In the silence the only sounds were the dogs' panting and the creak of the toboggans on the snow crystals. From time to time we would jump off our toboggans and jog for a while, adding the muffled sound of our mukluks pounding the snow followed shortly afterwards by our heavy breathing.

Then coming around a bend in the river, we saw a well-used trail leading up the riverbank to where a canvas tent was pitched. A lazy curl of smoke was coming from the stovepipe jutting out from the front of the tent. A frenzy of barking dogs soon heralded our arrival and Paul Koe stuck his head out of the tent before emerging, his eyes screwed up against the daylight. He told us that he and his partner Richard had been up all night hunting muskrat, and we could see the heap of skinned carcasses lying by the cold remains of a fire where the two young men had sat skinning their catch. We learned that John Itsi had just left their camp that morning and so we should have a good trail to follow.

True enough, a fresh dog team trail led away from the camp, and after wishing the boys good hunting, we started off along the trail, the dogs picking up speed again as they sensed another team somewhere ahead. We had decided to make camp at about four-thirty so we would have time to set our tent, gather brush and firewood and make ourselves comfortable for the night. But it turned out that the banks of the river were too high for us to climb and we were forced to keep travelling, hoping that there would be a suitable place around the next bend or the next. Then as we came around a bend of the river, looking eagerly along the bank for a low spot, we spied a small cabin. Jim Vittrekwa stood in the doorway, surrounded by what seemed like a horde of little children. When a woman's voice suddenly shouted, "You kids come back in here and shut the door!" I recognized the voice of Jim's wife, Ellen, and I smiled because she was usually a very quiet woman. I didn't know she had such a powerful voice! Reluctantly the children went back inside and Jim shut the door behind them.

"If you don't want to make camp," he said, "there are some more cabins about three kilometres from here. It's Andrew's place and there is probably room there for you there." Andrew Kunnizzi was a very respected elder from Fort McPherson and one of the neatest trappers I had met.

Thanking Jim, we called out to our now rather reluctant dogs and got them motivated to start a slow trot along the trail. "I think it would have been a bit crowded in there!" Shane called to me. "I didn't fancy sleeping with all of those kids crawling over me." I waved my agreement and we both then lapsed into silence as we travelled on in the waning light. We didn't have to worry about being caught out in the dark because at this time of the year it never did get completely dark, which is why the Gwich'in did their muskrat trapping during the night when it was cooler and the trails firmer. Within two months the ice that we were travelling on would have melted, the rivers and lakes would have open water on them, ducks, geese, swans and loons would be busy looking for their mates and the sun would be shining twenty-four hours a day. However, this knowledge did not make me feel any warmer as we headed into a cold north wind, and I began to worry that the people we were hoping to visit had all moved on. It was comforting to know that the few we had already seen were healthy because if any of them had been at all ill, they would have been demanding pills. But once again it came to me that living out in the bush, even in some of these pretty primitive camps, seemed to make both old and young thrive. It was always heartening to see lively youngsters with rosy cheeks, some of them as brown as could be after being outside under the brilliant springtime sun.

In a very short time we arrived at Andrew's place where three neat cabins stood on a patch of high ground. No one was there, but one of the cabins was open and we made ourselves at home. Lighting a fire in the stove and putting snow in the kettle to begin melting was the most important thing. Then taking the dogs out of harness, tying them up and feeding them were our next chores. They shook themselves, ate their food rapidly, and turning around several times sank onto their beds of spruce branches with what sounded like a sigh.

We didn't get an early start the next morning as Shane wanted to make a few repairs to his toboggan brake. While he did this, I made breakfast, then we loaded up and were on our way again. By noon we had reached Abe Koe's cabin, and while Shane chatted to Abe, his wife, Rosemary, asked me to look at her baby. The infant was all wrapped up in a swing crib suspended about shoulder-high in the corner of the cabin. These swings were quite innovative. A blanket was folded over two parallel ropes and pinned to form a hammock, and the ropes were held apart by pieces of wood at the foot and head of where the baby was to lie. The swing was then hung across the corner of a room so that from time to time it could be given a gentle push to pacify the baby.

Rosemary lifted her baby out of the swing while she was telling me that he was covered in a rash. When she undressed him, I could see the rash plainly. "Do you keep him in the swing all day?" I asked as I pulled out my stethoscope and warmed it by the stove.

"Most of the time. I bring him out to feed and change him, that's all."

I listened to the baby's chest and looked in his ears, and he seemed happy enough, not even worried by this bearded stranger handling him. In fact, he was more interested in the stethoscope, which made it difficult to hear any sensitive sounds, until Rosemary held his hands. I used a rectal thermometer to take his temperature and that made him squirm a bit, but his temperature was normal.

"I think all he has is a heat rash," I told her, "because he's getting too hot up there in the swing. Don't wrap him up too much during the daytime and just let him lie on your bed. He'll be okay there as long as you don't leave him alone." She seemed relieved to know that her baby didn't have some infectious disease, and I left her to talk to Abe while I washed the thermometer and my hands with a few medicated towelettes.

After we left the camp, we had been travelling on the river for less than two hours when we came to Fred Snowshoe's camp. Fred was out trapping but his wife was there with three small children,

and after I had fastened up my lead dog in the front and the toboggan at the back so that the team would not go on without me, I went
in to see them. Shane fastened his dogs behind mine before following me inside.

Sarah was a bright young mother and looked after her family
well but she reported that although two of the children were fine, the
youngest had scared her the previous night. "She had a convulsion and
her eyes went up and she seemed to go stiff for a short while."

When I examined the small infant, all I could find was a moderately elevated temperature. She did not seem to be very ill, but
the symptoms Sarah described could be quite serious. I was concerned that in all the cabins the wood stoves were crammed tight
with wood at night so by midnight the temperature soared. Then
by about three or four in the morning the wood had burned up
and the temperature plummeted. Babies who were well wrapped
up in the evening sweltered in the heat and then cooled rapidly
later on.

I checked the baby to make sure that there were no obvious signs
of meningitis, but she showed no distress as I moved her about. Then
because Sarah was a knowledgeable mother and would listen to my
advice, I told her to bathe her baby in warm water and give her some
infant fever medication at regular intervals as long as the fever per-
sisted. She didn't need a thermometer for this. As a good mother, she
knew the difference between her child being feverish or just plain
hot. She said that if it happened again, she would get her husband
to take them to the village, but she really didn't want to go unless it
was necessary because this was the best time for ratting and they depended on it for their income. I could understand her predicament
and knew that she would do the best thing for her family.

Shane and I carried on along the trail, and it came to me that
perhaps Shane wasn't getting to speak to many people because I
always seemed to get in there first, but at least he was seeing where
and how the people lived and I guessed that this was all part of "being on patrol." I noticed that he asked about the trapping and what

the weather had been like, and I am sure his friendly manner was not a threat to anyone.

We passed some old buildings high up on a riverbank, some of which looked as though they were about to fall into the river as it had eaten its way into the muddy bank. I told Shane that this was the Harrisons' mink farm and that I had stayed in this cabin a couple of years or so earlier when Muriel and I, with two teacher friends, Mike and Bett Wiggins, had gone by dog team from Fort McPherson to Aklavik during the Easter holidays. "This place was abandoned even back then." We tied the dogs up at the bottom of the bank and scrambled to the top to have a look around then made a small fire and ate lunch, though rather late as it was almost four o'clock. It was still very light. Returning to the river, we shouted to the dogs who once again got to their feet rather reluctantly and shook themselves. After our inactivity we were now beginning to feel the cold, and to add to our discomfort the north wind had started to blow and a fine snow was drifting over the trail we were following. By six we were feeling solidly frozen and were thankful to see a small log cabin ahead of us with thick smoke pouring out of the chimney.

"Johnny Lenny's cabin!" I shouted to Shane through frozen lips. I had fond memories of staying at the Lennys' cabin when they had fed our starving—well, hungry anyway—little party with freshly baked bread laden with butter and cheese, followed by cups of freshly brewed coffee.

Johnny had a remarkable camp. His woodpile was almost as high as the house, eliminating the need to hunt for wood during the winter, because he harvested his vital wood supply from along the riverbank in summer, hauling it to his cabin by boat. The cabin interior was painted and clean, the floor scrubbed almost white, and everything was in its place.

Johnny and his wife now came to the rescue of Shane and me with an offer of fresh coffee, then after peering outside and seeing that a heavy snowstorm had started, he invited us to stay in his old cabin, an offer we were more than glad to accept. Radio Station

CHAK from Inuvik was broadcasting the weather report on his battery-powered radio, and I was startled to hear that there was a wind chill factor of minus fifty-five degrees (C) in Inuvik, just eighty kilometres north of the Lennys' camp. No wonder Shane and I had felt half-frozen!

With Johnny's assistance we tied the dogs and fed them and Shane brought in one of the sets of dog harness to repair. Star, one of William's dogs, had chewed through a strap, probably while we were at Harrison's mink farm. After a supper of moose steak and potatoes, Johnny came to our cabin and marked our maps with the route we should take to the Husky Channel and back to the Peel River. He also knew where most of the other cabins were located and we marked them on our map as well. The next morning, after a leisurely breakfast of bacon and eggs, a royal feast considering we were so far out in the bush, we sat and talked with the Lennys, who told us that they really enjoyed having company because they saw so few people.

After the snowstorm the temperature rose to minus twelve degrees (C), and we knew that if it got any warmer, the snow would be wet and the dogs would have a tough time working in it. We left at mid-morning in a small gale, the fine snow blowing into our faces and finding its way into the neck of my parka. It was a relief when at last we turned east toward a group of old cabins, which stood looking out over the junction of two rivers. At one time there had been a store here that was referred to as Laing's place, but Knute Laing had died quite awhile ago. For several years after that an old man named Ed Rydstedt had looked after the buildings and the few supplies that remained, but as sometimes happens to people who live absolutely alone for too long in an isolated place, he became a little strange and was said to raise pups so he could eat them. Finally he was taken to a care facility in Aklavik. No one lived there now and we stopped for a few minutes to look around but did not go into any of the buildings.

Afterwards we turned our dogs and set off down Phillip's Channel (known locally as the Neyuck channel), and following a trail from the river we came to a portage beside a creek where there was lots of overflow. On one side of the trail, a lake was either thawing or had a natural spring in it and the water from it was draining into the channel. Luckily, a huge natural ice bridge had formed nearby and we crossed over this very gingerly.

At the mouth of the channel we had been following we came out onto the Husky River where Johnny Semple's cabin was located. A number of Dall sheepskins were on the roof and inside the cabin, and it was obvious that this was his base camp for sheep hunting, but he wasn't there. We went in to have lunch and make a fire to boil water for tea, but the stove had been made from an old forty-five-gallon barrel, and when the kettle took forever to boil, we ended up balancing it on the burning wood and were finally able to make our pot of tea. Of course, we then had to wait for the tea to cool down enough that we could drink it, but it was good to feel that scalding liquid go into our insides and feel the heat radiating out.

We travelled on the Husky River as far as Sheep Creek where the sheep were hunted, and then as there was no trail, I snowshoed ahead for two hours with Shane urging the two teams to follow me. We finally came to another cabin where the lone occupant, a young man known as John Alex, was stretching rats. He explained that he was getting quite a few muskrats and he expected to be staying at the cabin for a few more days. The cabin belonged to old John Roberts but he had retired after working for the game warden for a number of years. He had not been down to his cabin for a long time and it had begun to fall apart.

Young Alex said there was a good trail from his place to Johnny Charlie's cabin, which was only about six points on the river further on. Unfortunately, we found the trail completely obliterated, and after counting at least a dozen points, we gave up counting. Two and a half hours later we arrived with very tired dogs at Johnny Charlie's empty cabin. Next door was a much smaller cabin where his father, old Alfred Tetlichi, had lived during the ratting season, and it would

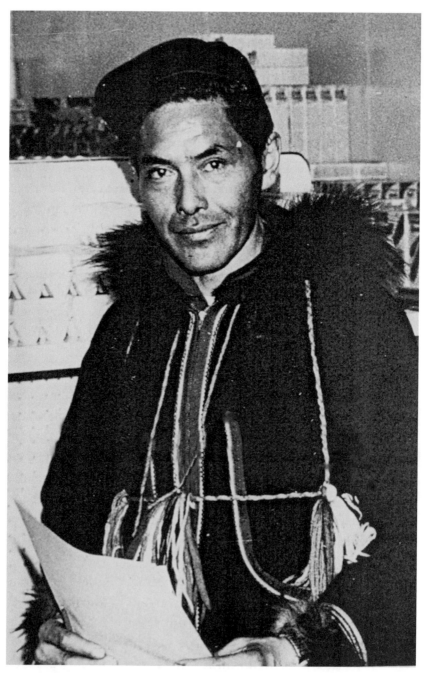

Johnny Charlie had a cabin and trapping trail on the Husky River.
FRANK DUNN PHOTO.

have been large enough for Shane and me, but as there was no stove we stayed the night in Johnny's cabin.

We were on the trail again by late morning, but after going no more than a kilometre we realized that we must be on Johnny's trapping trail as it wandered from one small lake to the next. Retracing our steps to the cabin, we searched for another trail and finding none, began following the river again, breaking trail for four hours before arriving at Mary Wilson's cabin. She explained that the portage trail we had missed started right behind Johnny's cabin and would have saved us two hours! Mary already had a houseful of visitors, with Lydia Elias and Bertha Francis and her family staying there, but she offered us some tea and bannock and we went into the cabin and talked with the women. They all teased us and laughed because we had taken the long route from Johnny's, then they told us that all of their menfolk had gone hunting caribou at Sheep Creek and they didn't know when they would get back. They described the next portages to us in detail and kept telling us, along with a lot of laughter, not to get lost this time. Following their instructions, which were very precise, we came to Joe and Beatrice Jerome's camp at five that afternoon, and Beatrice told us that her menfolk were all away hunting caribou, too, but that Old Chief Johnny Kay's cabin was just a short distance away on Caribou Creek and he and his wife were there.

Johnny Kay and his wife, Edith, were a quiet couple, and their aristocratic bearing showed why they were venerated by all the Gwich'in people. They had a quiet dignity in the way they spoke and moved, and they were extremely polite and asked us if we would share some tea and doughnuts that Edith had made shortly before we arrived.

After Shane had retied some babiche that had broken on his toboggan, we took our leave from the Kays, and Johnny said quietly, "Thank you for visiting us." He had been a special constable and guide for the Royal North West Mounted Police and had travelled thousands of kilometres by dog team, and though now in his eighties, he still drove a team, as did his wife who was not much younger.

And here he was saying "Thank you" to a pair of relatively soft and untried white men. But I was sure Shane had found speaking to old Johnny Kay especially satisfying, because the old man represented a long-gone part of the force's history, a romantic and picturesque era that was palpable as we spoke to this almost regal man at his log cabin with his husky dogs in the snowy background.

We followed a portage that took us back to the Husky River and found a few cabins beside the creek that entered the Husky River here. Sarah Debastien was staying here with the two young sons of Edward Blake, and unlike many of the Gwich'in women, she was not shy and could hold her own in a conversation with anyone, anywhere. Her grandfather, the first Edward Blake, had also been a member of the Royal North West Mounted Police; perhaps she had inherited her forthright manner from him. She told us that her husband, Ernie Debastien, had recently driven from Fort McPherson to the cabin on a snowmobile, so the trail should be broken for us. As everyone was healthy and busy with muskrat trapping, we didn't stay long, leaving at eight in the evening.

Following the snowmobile track for a short distance, we joined the main dog team trail that we had travelled at the beginning of our journey. We now had made a complete circle in the Delta and before long we caught sight of the village lights ahead. After unloading and then feeding the dogs, I gave them a good pat and a rub over their ears. They had taken me over good trails, bad trails and no trails at all, but had worked well, finally bringing me home. Muriel had already gone to bed but was still awake. She got up and made me some supper while I cleaned up. When the phone rang, it was Shane to say that he had taken the dogs back to William. "They were so tired that they were not interested in eating at first, but William said he would see they were all right so I came home. We'll see you tomorrow."

Shane and I had both learned a lot about the people of the Mackenzie Delta on our trip to the rat camps. We wondered how long this way of life would continue in the fast-changing North, but we had experienced it as it was, and it was good for us.

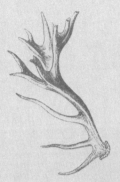

SOMETIME IN THE PAST THE FAMILY of Johnny and Edith Kay had shortened their name from Kayukavitchuk—or as relatives in Old Crow spelled it, Kyikavichik—because not many white people could pronounce it and tended to use just the part of the name they could pronounce.

Gwich'in personal names have almost disappeared from use and a lot of the original names have been changed to European names. Some have just been corrupted from the original. The name Itsi came from Edze, meaning "ear." Other names were equally descriptive; for example, the surname Drymeat was used until the early fifties at which time that family's younger people started using their father's Christian name of Peter as their surname. In the mid- to late-1800s, the names of some patriarchs were preserved in their English form but not in the Gwich'in vocabulary, and the anthropologist Richard Slobodin cites names such as "Painted Face's Father." Not surprisingly, his son was called "Painted Face," and I had to wonder what the father was called before his son was born. Painted Face had one brother named "Caribou Boy" and another named "Small Nipples," although the latter was also known as Charles Francis. Both Painted Face and Caribou Boy were killed in a skirmish with a raiding Eskimo party. Charles Francis had a son who was called Tsik or "Slim" Francis. "Tame Thomas" and Lucy Martin "Cuts Birch" had two boys, Peter and Julius. As the family lines descended, so the Gwich'in names seemed to go into obscurity.

CHAPTER THIRTEEN

BEING INVOLVED IN THE COMMUNITY WAS an important part of Muriel's and my own enjoyment of our time working in the North, and spring was probably the most exciting time to be there. The air was full of expectation and long before the ice broke up, we would see ducks flying overhead. One spring as I was travelling by dogsled to Arctic Red River, I was surprised to see two ducks flying close overhead and then over the snow and ice, down the lake. These were the really "early birds"!

As the snow melted, the runoff formed muddy pools in the village, but the ice on the river stayed firm and the people continued to travel to and from their camps quite easily. In fact, the deep snow on the river had packed down and travelling was much easier, but they preferred to travel at night when it was a bit cooler and some of the pools of water lying on the ice had frozen again. On both sides of the river ice, the melting water ran in channels so that, when you crossed the river, you had to wade through fifteen centimetres of running water to reach the ice. At first I thought this was rather scary, but as with anything you do numerous times without any bad effects, I soon hardly thought about it as I crossed the river with Mary Firth to check her muskrat traps on some of the small lakes on her trapline.

Mary and I would struggle up the riverbank on the west side of the Peel, slipping on the icy mud until we reached the top, and then

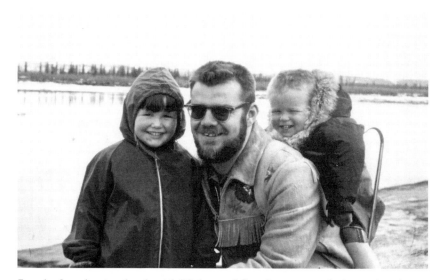

I rushed to the riverbank with Helen and Stephen to watch the ice break up.

we donned our snowshoes and walked along her trapline trail. At the first lake, which was about half a kilometre wide, the traps were set in the weedy push-up houses toward its centre, and we had only walked a few metres onto the ice when there was a sound of muffled thunder and the whole surface of the lake seemed to sink. I froze in my tracks, and Mary hesitated a moment before laughing and telling me, "It's okay. The ice is still good. That happens when the snow underneath gets soft, and when someone steps on the icy top, it just goes down a bit,"

This was comforting news, and I was glad that Mary was with me because otherwise I would have been reluctant to carry on, even though it had happened to me before. But every time I experienced it, I immediately stopped to wonder *What if...?* I crouched to scrape the snow from the surface of the ice and saw that it was dry and had no overflow at all.

Mary's husband, William, had told me that people in the bush made a practice of carrying long, thin poles on their shoulders when they crossed a lake or a river for the first time in the fall, so that if they stepped onto a patch of thin ice or into a hole and broke through, they would have something to hang onto that would help get them out again. And if they were with a companion, he or she could grasp one end of the pole and pull the person from the water.

❄ ❄ ❄

Preparations for the spring ice breakup were fun to watch. A tripod was set up in the middle of the Peel River opposite the Hudson's Bay manager's house and on top of the tripod a flag of some description was fastened so that it could easily be seen from the shore. The Community Club then started an ice breakup pool wherein the participants had to guess the time of day that the ice would move, and the time guessed had to be right down to the minute. This always started the "I remember when" stories circulating, and the old-timers would sit visiting in houses all over the village, giving a history of ice breakups they had witnessed. Some with nothing better to do would sit in the hot sun on the dry grass in front of the Bay house, smoking and talking but keeping their eyes on the marker. Every time Muriel and I left the nursing station to go on home visits, we would check the flag on the tripod as we walked along the top of the riverbank and past the church and the graveyard. And people we met along the way or at the homes we visited would ask, "Anything moving yet?"

One afternoon, shortly after the children went back to school after lunch, the wail of the village fire alarm sounded and we knew that this meant just one thing. The ice had broken and the flag was moving! I felt sorry for the teachers in school who now had to control excited children who wanted to know immediately who had won the ice pool. Like most of the people who were free to do so, we walked over to the riverbank and watched as a dark crack in the ice widened and the marker moved down the river on a big cake of ice. More cracks appeared and the ice gathered momentum. Even from the top of the bank we could hear the grinding of the floes as they heaved and churned against each other, pushed by an ever-increasing flow of muddy river water.

One breakup Muriel and I walked our two small children down to the dock to get a closer look at the ice, and as we stared out across the river, I had the distinct impression that we were moving upriver and that the ice was standing still. I shook my head and everything returned to normal. Some of the smaller ice floes had been turned upside down in the maelstrom and revealed their unevenly polished undersides where the constantly flowing silty water had smoothed them. Then, as the big floes were pushed on end, we could see how the ice was made up of multiple ice candles that broke away with a tinkling sound. The whole process kept us spellbound, and for some reason it was exciting and at the same time scary as we saw the power of the water and ice, which could shear large trees from the riverbank and crush them like matchwood. But I was always sorry to see the ice go out, disappointed that I could not travel on it anymore.

As the floes from further up the river came by, it was as if they each carried an untold story—a section of dog team trail on one, several prints etched in the melting snow showed that wolves had crossed another. Some large animal had sat or lain down on a section of one of the floes, but we assumed it was long gone by the time the ice broke up because most animals seem to have an uncanny sense of the safety of the ice. They never seem to cross too early in the fall or too late in the springtime, though one trapper told me of seeing a moose frozen in a lake. The trapper had seen an unusual snow-covered shape in the middle of the lake and, investigating, found that it was a young moose that had frozen in the water. By the time he found it any weakness in the ice had disappeared, so he assumed the moose had tried crossing when the shore ice was firm but possibly a spring or gas bubbles from rotting vegetation had weakened that particular section of lake.

For a couple of days after breakup the ice would continue to flow, and then it would slow right down. "The Mackenzie won't be breaking up yet," William Firth told us knowingly. "So the water will be backing up down at the Mouth of the Peel. That water can come up pretty quick," he continued, "and sometimes people have to stay in their scows if it gets too deep." I had seen the high water marks at the Harrisons' mink farm during a winter dog team trip. Their cabin, which was on a bank ten metres above the river's surface, had a high water line two metres up the wall inside the house. That would have been scary! Because of the frequent spring flooding of the Peel River at Aklavik and the consequent land erosion, in 1953 the federal government tried to move the village to a site known as East Three, sixty kilometres to the east, but the location was too far from traditional hunting and trapping territory. Five years later government offices were moved to the new site, now christened Inuvik, but most of the real northerners stayed on in Aklavik and put up with the flooding.

As soon as the snow had melted on the sandbar in front of Fort McPherson, the ducks landed by the hundreds. Next came the geese, and between their honking and the ducks' constant squawking, it was like bedlam all day and all night. Whenever someone walked down the riverbank toward them, the whirring of countless wings was like a strong wind as they whirled around and came down again to land and start their haggling all over again.

One evening when we were having supper with Constable Frank Dunn and his wife, Janje, Frank asked if I would like to go duck hunting with him. I immediately accepted, not that I wanted to shoot ducks but because Frank was going to use his homemade wooden boat that had an airplane engine with a large prop attached to the stern. It was decided that we would go the following day, so after supper, and because the Dunns also had two small children, Sherry and Peter, we took our two children home quite early. As Muriel undressed two-year-old Stephen to put him into his pyjamas, some pieces of cutlery fell out of his coverall bib. I picked up several knives and forks and with a laugh told Muriel that they were all stamped with the RCMP logo! "I didn't know we were raising such a young kleptomaniac, but fancy pinching them from the police of all people!" But we couldn't understand how or when he had stuck them into his clothes because he had not been given any large cutlery.

"Frank is going to be watching my every move tomorrow in case he thinks it is a family failing," I said as we tucked the children into their beds. I returned the cutlery to Janje when I went to meet Frank

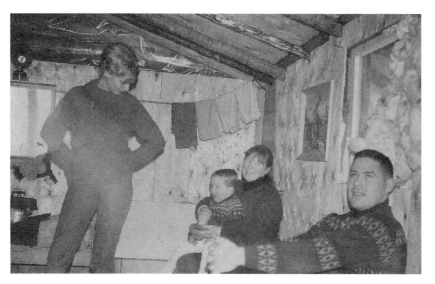

Frank and Janje Dunn visiting me, my wife, and son Stephen.

the next morning and she said that they hadn't even missed them.

Frank's boat had been christened the *Scoot* and it was as noisy as an airplane. With its two large plywood rudders fastened to the propeller frame, it could travel easily over water and sandbar or ice and snow. There was just enough room in it for Frank, myself and a barrel of gas. Frank took his shotgun, showing me that he also had a couple of high-powered slugs just in case there was an early-rising bear out after some duck meat. We blasted down to the river and over a small slough and onto a long sandbar. The engine made so much noise I couldn't see a duck for miles, but we scooted around until we were getting a bit short of gas. We didn't get any ducks and I think I lost a segment of my hearing, but we had a great time!

❄   ❄   ❄

Gradually the number of ice floes that came by decreased, but as they did so, the water rose higher and higher by the hour. By this time the sandbar that had been covered with water fowl had disappeared under the fast-rising water, and as the water increased in velocity, it began to wash away all the debris accumulated over nine months of winter, plus trees and bushes from a hundred kilometres of riverbank. To try to navigate a scow in the river at this time would have been disastrous.

Once the excitement of the ice breakup had subsided, we were faced with the realities of springtime. Overflowing and flooded outhouses and household garbage that had been blown about by the cold winds of winter and then covered with snow—out of sight and out of mind—now floated about on the numerous pools of melted snow and ice. Roads that had been hard-packed and firm to drive on just weeks earlier were now a sticky, gooey mess, and any attempt to cross them left us with feet of lead as a steadily increasing load of mud stuck to our boots. Fortunately, wooden sidewalks had been constructed on both sides of the road, so if we kept to one side we could make it from the nursing station to the school relatively unscathed.

One year as the water in the Peel River subsided and float planes were able to make their way to Fort McPherson again, we were pleased to learn that a couple of popular singers from Outside were going to come to the village and put on a show. Ian and Sylvia Tyson were stars of radio (and of television down south where it was available) and we all looked forward to meeting them. The place where the plane was to land was several metres from the dry bank, and we could see that the expanse of thick gooey mud lying between would be impassable. However, I thought if we put some planks down, our guests would be able to get across the mud unscathed.

On the day of the event I managed to manoeuvre myself into a position where I could be the first to greet them when they disembarked. I walked down the plank as they clambered down from the plane then stepped from the float onto the plank. It was only then that I realized there would not be enough room for them to pass me, so I courteously stepped off the board and immediately felt myself sinking up to my knees in the thick mud. When Sylvia reached me, my head was just about level with her waist, and as I held out my hand in greeting, she grasped it thankfully to prevent herself from losing her balance and then walked on while I continued to stand there with a sinking feeling. Ian followed behind her and all I could do was offer him the same support. He probably wondered why this person with the very short legs was standing patiently in the mud! After they climbed into a waiting vehicle and were driven to the village, I struggled out of my rubber boots, then kneeling on the muddy plank, struggled to free them from nearly a metre of gumbo. Covered in mud, I squished my way home to clean up, thinking that Sir Walter Raleigh, who according to tradition placed his cape over a puddle so that Queen Elizabeth wouldn't wet her feet, never knew how easy he had it!

※　※　※

Each spring when all the snow had finally gone, it was time for Fort McPherson's annual cleanup, and nearly everyone except possibly the really aged and infirm would set about raking up the sawdust and bits of bark that had accumulated during a winter's worth of cutting and splitting firewood. As sweet-smelling woodsmoke from the many smouldering yard fires drifted over the village, it was quite pleasant to walk along the main street and see an improvement in the general looks of the village day by day. The Indian agent organized a truck to pick up the plastic bags filled with paper, cans and other garbage that the villagers had collected and had them taken to the dump on the northern outskirts of the village.

One spring, while most of the village was cleaning up the accumulated garbage, the staff at the Northern Canada Power Corporation and the RCMP decided that they should remove an old shack that was half a kilometre to the south of the main village. But this was no ordinary shack. It had been used to store explosives, and to prevent inquisitive persons from breaking into it, plainly written on the front of the building in large red letters was a sign warning "Danger, Dynamite!"

The decision to remove it had come after a worker had made a routine inspection of the shack and then remarked to the RCMP corporal that he had seen some nitroglycerine running across the floorboards and hadn't hung around to investigate further. As it was too dangerous to try to move the building, they prepared to blow it up where it was, and arrangements were made to do this in the middle of an afternoon when the schoolchildren were in school so that there would be little chance of a curious onlooker being hurt. The road that went past the shack and led to a pump house was blocked on the appointed day, but for safety reasons the event was not publicized. This was a well-intentioned decision, but to a small, quiet community that only heard large noises from shotguns, the resulting boom that shook the ground—and I'm sure rattled every window north of 60—caused some consternation. Muriel and I were catching up on our paperwork when the explosion occurred at the opposite end of the village, and we felt the ground shake and our windows rattled so much I feared they would break. As it was doubtful that we were being bombed, we concluded that a boiler must have blown up in the generating plant and feared there could be a lot of injuries. William dashed in looking scared and asked us what had happened, but as we couldn't tell him anything, he went off to find out. When the fire siren failed to sound and no one called for our medical services, we began to relax. A short time later William returned with a smile on his face and recounted the story of the dynamite shack. All we could think of was that it sure made a thorough job of the cleanup of the shack.

❆　❆　❆

Spring brought out the insect population, and besides myriads of mosquitoes and blackflies, there were bees, wasps, spiders, horseflies and bluebottles to prevent us from really enjoying the season. Dragonflies feasted on the abundance of mosquitoes and other insects, but even though they were known to eat a lot of them in a day, they didn't seem to make much difference to the overall insect population. The environment section of Health and Welfare sent us some small cubes of gel-covered mosquito insecticide, which we were instructed to put into any standing pools of water. The cubes were supposed to melt in the heat of the day, spreading an oily substance on the surface of the water, killing the mosquito larvae. But someone had forgotten to do his research on the temperature of Fort McPherson's pools in the springtime because when we went around to check on our handiwork a few days later, the same little cubes were still floating on the water as solid as they were when we dropped them in.

Another springtime event—which when I think back on it makes me shudder—was a procedure using a gas-powered fogger. Muriel and I would sit on the back of a pickup truck that was driven all around the village while clouds of insecticide were pumped out, so when viewed from a distance, the village looked as though it was shrouded in an early fog. For some reason, it was thought that this should be the nurses' job because mosquito bites caused impetigo and other diseases.

Mosquitoes spoiled many a planned walk. Shortly after we arrived in Fort McPherson, we almost gave up on walks after one foray when it had seemed as if the mosquitoes had only waited for us to get into the bush before attacking. We fled back to the nursing station as fast as we could, and when we pulled off our clothes, we discovered that those varmints had already found their way through layers of clothing to our warm English blood.

But there was a greater peril. "Going out" was the Gwich'in term for going to the bathroom because in the sixties the majority did not have bathrooms and had to "go out" either to their outdoor toilets when in the village or to the nearest bush if they were at camp. But "going out" when you were out in the bush in the summertime was a hurried affair if you didn't want to end up with a multitude of bites on your rear end, and I well remember Muriel having to treat one teacher who had come to Fort McPherson on a canoe trip from Aklavik. She had acquired some blackfly bites that had become infected and made sitting down very uncomfortable for her.

It took us a few years of visiting summer fish camps out in the bush before we observed that the Gwich'in did not seem to be as troubled as we were by biting insects. At one camp I was suddenly aware that I was standing there waving my arms around like a windmill out of control, swatting at the attacking mosquitoes and blackflies, while our hosts, an elderly couple with wrinkled brown skin, sat sedately on some logs, now and again picking off a mosquito that had landed on a forearm or a cheek. It was then that I realized I was pumping up a real head of steam as I thrashed around and the resulting sweaty aroma was evidently irresistible to the insects. It took a lot of control to emulate these bush-wise people, and every spring I had to relearn their ways. However, we did discover that after the initial outburst of insects in the springtime, either we became accustomed to them or they declined in number, and by late August we could go outside without daubing insect dope on all the exposed areas of skin.

CHAPTER FOURTEEN

As the daylight increased, we looked forward to the phenomenon of the midnight sun. One summer, as it got closer to the time, Helen Sullivan, the Bay manager's wife, called to ask if we would like to bring the children and join her and Dave for a wiener roast to celebrate the midnight sun. She hurriedly explained that we wouldn't be having it at midnight because Dave had to work the next day and she knew that our children would not be able to stay awake that long. We all went down to the sandbar, made a fire big enough to roast wieners and marshmallows and we sat around and talked, enjoying the sunlight. The sun was high even though it was nine o'clock and it would not set for another month. There was not a fly or mosquito to be seen, ducks quacked on the muddy shoreline and the air was warm and fresh. Afterwards we took the children home and tucked them into their beds. To them these things they were witnessing were not unusual; they were just a part of their normal life.

It was a few weeks later that both Muriel and I were awakened at three in the morning by some crashes and bangs and then the sound of Stephen's laughter. When we opened the door to the children's bedroom, they looked at us and laughed. They were having a great time throwing their pillows at each other. We looked outside where it was clear and sunny and realized that to the children it was daylight so it must be time to get up.

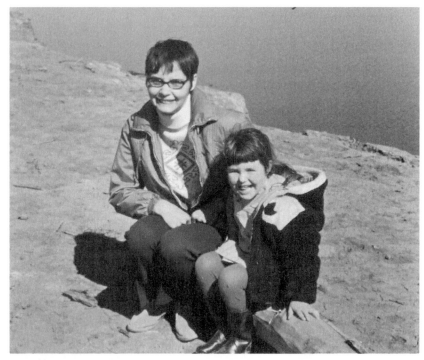

Two Helens, Helen Sullivan and Helen Billington, enjoy the spring air on the Peel River.

Muriel put the children to bed again and I found a box of tinfoil and taped two layers of it over the window. By the time I finished, the room was dark and the children were lying down. We sat in the kitchen to make sure that they didn't get up again and when we checked on them half an hour later they were both asleep again. Unfortunately, we were wide awake and when we went back to bed, the daylight in our room kept us awake until it was time to get up.

Sometimes when we were called out to a medical emergency in the middle of the night we would see small children playing outside. This was not really surprising because so many of the adults were trapping at night when it was cooler that a good percentage of the village had their days and nights reversed. I can remember being very annoyed when the nursing station buzzer sounded at three in the morning, and when I went to the door, I discovered it was a man

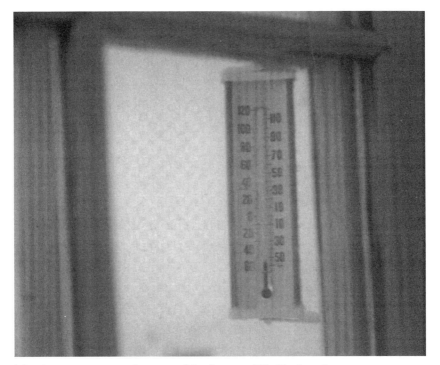

The thermometer reads minus fifty degrees (C). Earlier that morning it was below minus sixty!

asking for Band-Aids. To him it was the middle of the afternoon!

＊　＊　＊

The weather never failed to excite me. First thing in the morning I would open the curtains on the west side of the building and peer at the thermometer and then at the sky to see just what we had actually got and whether the various forecasts we had heard in any way matched the reality.

However, in the years that we spent in the Mackenzie Delta we found that certain dates gave us an indication of what weather to expect. Halloween would see snow on the ground that would last until the following year. Christmastime would be dark, very cold and—without exception—white. By Easter the sun would be glaring on the sun and ice, and the temperature would generally be in the minus thirties (C) and by July everywhere would be very, very muddy.

But the weather at any time of the year could change rapidly from one extreme to the other. I had experienced this one August when travelling up the Peel River in a speedboat, enjoying the hot breeze on my bare skin. Several hours later on the return journey, black clouds had rolled in, the temperature had plummeted and by the time we reached the village there was fifteen centimetres of snow on the ground and I thought that I had frostbitten my toes! Our vegetable garden that had been so promising was now a sea of wilting leaves, although the carrot tops still bravely stuck their tops up through the snow.

When it became really hot during the summertime, I longed to go for a swim, but the river was far too cold and the lakes were not accessible, and even if they had been, they would have been cold, as they sit on permafrost. However, one of the RCMP constables told me that he had a wetsuit, and as he was my size he offered to let me try it in the river. I had never worn a wetsuit before and I had great fun getting into it and by the time it was on I was really looking forward to jumping into some cold water. As I waded out into the muddy river, clouds of mosquitoes followed me but not one got through. I could feel the water creep up my legs as I walked deeper, and it was a strange sensation—cold for the first few seconds then it seemed to warm up and within minutes I was swimming and enjoying it thoroughly. I swam over to the other side of the river, just so I could say that I had, and then started back. But when I checked on the shoreline, I saw that it was zipping by at quite a fast rate and then suddenly it came to me: it's not zipping by! It's *me* that's zipping by! I didn't want to get caught in the current and end up in the Delta so I swam as hard as I could to the shallows and then walked back along the muddy shore to where Muriel was waiting. The experience was one of those things that I felt had to be done; it was exciting, a bit scary in a way, and that one dip in the river satisfied me.

❄ ❄ ❄

Canoes were common in the Mackenzie Delta in the sixties because the Gwich'in found them easy to portage between the many lakes

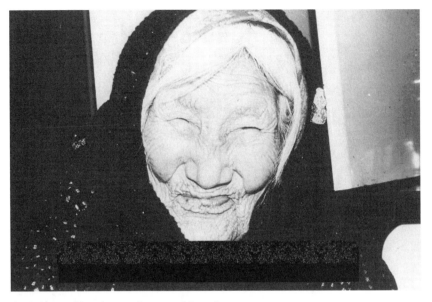

Old Annie Vaneltsi with a twinkle in her eye. FRANK DUNN PHOTO.

when they were muskrat trapping in the springtime as well as convenient to use for checking their fishnets on the river in summer. I had borrowed William Firth's canoe a few times and had quickly learned that travelling by canoe with the current was fast and easy, though on sharp bends in the River I had to take care to stay away from overhanging banks where the permafrost had been undermined. In fact, many of the riverbanks looked as though they were in imminent danger of collapse.

Late one beautiful evening when the midnight sun was low on the northern horizon, as frequently occurred when it was light for twenty-four hours, Muriel and I did not feel tired, and the still, calm waters of the Peel beckoned to us. We asked Mary Firth to come to the nursing station to sit with our children, who were asleep in bed, and to be there for Old Annie Vaneltsi, at ninety-six years the oldest person in the village, who was recovering from pneumonia. It was close to midnight but Mary said she didn't mind; she would sit with Annie and do some beadwork. "Take your .22 and shoot some rats for me," she said.

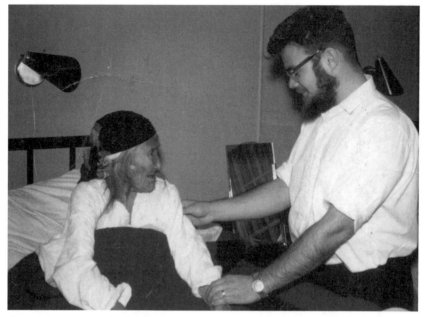

Annie recovered from pneumonia in the nursing station. She was very patient with me!

We showed Mary how to use the radio and said if anything happened and we were needed to press the call button and we would answer immediately. Mobile radios and the early "walkie-talkies" were still rather cumbersome in the sixties, but the previous winter when we realized they could be very useful to us, we had sent to Acme Novelty Company in Edmonton and ordered two of them. We found that as long as there was a good line of sight, especially across water, they would transmit and receive reasonably well over a distance of two kilometres. Then one evening as I sat playing around with the multitude of channels that were available, not expecting to hear another voice because as far as I knew no one in the village had a comparable phone, I heard a voice quite distinctly. Curious, I turned up the volume and listened to what was being said. By some quirk of the atmosphere I had tuned into the Alaska radio-telephone system, and being somewhat bored, for a short time I listened in to private conversations before feeling guilty and changing stations. Fortunately, I didn't know where in Alaska the calls were originating and I didn't know the people involved, but sitting in an isolated settlement where there was no entertainment made it very tempting to tune in now and again!

Now I explained to Mary, "When we have paddled up the creek, I'll call you so you can see how the phone works and you can tell us if everything is okay." I showed her how to switch from the call button to the receive mode. We tried it out a few times in the nursing station and Mary seemed to understand what to do.

❄   ❄   ❄

Muriel and I dragged William's canoe down to the river and, pushing out from the dock, paddled up the river a short way before turning into the current. Then still paddling as though we were going up the river, we allowed the canoe to be swept down and across it so that we came to the mouth of the little creek opposite the village. As soon as we entered the creek, we were able to paddle in a leisurely manner. The water was high because of the spring freshet and we saw several muskrat swimming so I tried calling to them, making the kissing noise that Mary had said was either a distress or a mating call. Muriel said it was lucky for me that I wasn't a muskrat! I saw a large rabbit on the shore, and thinking it would go nicely in the pot, I took a shot at it, but to our surprise it was a lynx. He jumped high in the air when he heard the shot and then bounded away into the bush unharmed.

After paddling for half an hour we thought that we should call Mary to make sure that everything was okay and let her know where we were. I pressed the call button and waited. Nothing. I pressed it again and waited. Still nothing. I checked my batteries but they were brand new. It was probably nothing to worry about, but just in case something was happening, we turned around and paddled back. Within an hour we were walking into the nursing station.

Mary was sitting in the armchair doing beadwork and she looked up and smiled as we walked in.

"Everything okay?" I asked.

"Sure, Annie went to sleep a long time ago. After I made tea, she didn't even finish it! The children are both fast asleep."

"Did you hear the radiophone? We called you several times."

"Yes, it buzzed and made me jump," she said, pointing to where we had hung it by the window, "but I was shy to say anything so I left it."

This was typical of Mary and many of the women in Fort McPherson, who would sound so confident at times and then would fold into themselves with shyness or embarrassment at other times. When I had been on the trapline with Mary and she knew I would be taking her photograph, she would suddenly put up her hand, pull her headscarf down and giggle with embarrassment. Of course, she was missing some of her upper teeth, and when she was out working, she didn't put in her plate so maybe that was the cause of some of her photosensitivity.

After this failed episode with the radiophone, we asked the RCMP to keep one of our units at their office, but they said that there was no need. If anything happened, they would come and find us wherever we were. After phones were installed in the village we could just leave a phone number with William and a number on the clinic door.

❉ ❉ ❉

On several other occasions Muriel and I borrowed William Firth's canoe, and by paddling like demons we were able to cross the river and go up a small creek opposite the village where we hunted beaver and muskrat for Mary Firth and where we built a small cabin. One year as springtime gave way to summer, we noticed there was an abundance of wildflowers in that area, and we thought it would be nice to make a garden using local flora. We started collecting some of the plants that were just beginning to show, struggling up out of the few centimetres of soil that covered the permafrost, which was never more than fifteen centimetres below the surface. Then we remembered that we had seen wild lupines on a high bank on the west side of the river, their deep blue flowers contrasting sharply with the grey shale that surrounded them. Above them on top of the bank, small birch and spruce trees grew amid a profusion of willow bushes. Using William's canoe, Muriel and I paddled across the river then followed the shore for a short distance. As we got out and pulled the canoe high up on one of the few gravel beaches, the sun beat down on us, and we rested for a few minutes and shared a drink from the bottle of water we had brought with us.

"I think this is where the village used to be a long time ago," I said. William had pointed out the general direction to us a few weeks previously.

"It looks like a better spot than where the village is now," Muriel said, and pointing up at the high bank, she continued, "It's higher and the ground isn't as swampy as it is behind McPherson."

"Let's see if there are any signs of the old place," I suggested. We made enough noise climbing the hill, clattering through the bush and talking to each other that no self-respecting bear would have come close to us, but we really weren't thinking about bears. We were looking for signs of old cabins or even the stumps of trees to show that someone had been there but all we saw was an endless sea of thick bush.

"Look over there!" I pointed to a small depression in the hillside. "It's a grave! See the little picket fence around it—or what's left of it anyway." We pushed through the bush and gazed at a very old grave. The little picket fence with its sawn ends was still standing on two sides but the other two had rotted and collapsed. There was no marker evident and forest debris covered the top of the grave.

"I wonder who was buried here," Muriel said, and looking up through the canopy of trees, noticed that clouds were now scurrying across the sky. She shivered. "C'mon, it's getting colder. Let's go back and ask William who it was."

When we came down to the river, we saw that the sun was now covered by cloud and a north wind had sprung up, so we hurriedly pushed the canoe back into the water, stepped in and paddled for the opposite shore. The north wind whipped against the current and it was hard paddling against the waves so we were thankful to get ashore. But by the time we arrived at the door of William and Mary's house, the wind had died and the sun was shining again.

Mary came to the door and ushered us inside. "Oh, you both look so cold! You need some tea." And she went to the cupboard and brought out some freshly baked bannock to go with the tea.

"We wanted to ask you about the grave on the other side of the river," Muriel began just as William came in through the back door.

"What grave?" he asked, and we told him about our trip over the river and finding the old grave.

"There's no grave over there," he said, glancing at Mary.

She nodded in agreement. "Maybe it was just the roots of a tree that you saw."

"No, it definitely was a grave with an old picket fence round it just like you see in the church graveyard, only this one was really old and falling down."

"I don't know of any grave and I've never heard anyone talk about one either." William said, shaking his head.

"Well, we'll be going over there again in a day or two to get some lupines and I'll take some pictures to show you," I said, and we finished our tea and went home.

"That was really weird," I said, "and it was creepy when that wind came up and then just as fast died down again. Lucky we're not superstitious!"

It was another week before we had time to cross the river again. The weather was mild, there was no wind and the sun was shining. We landed on the same small beach and walked into the bush.

"Can you remember where it was?" Muriel asked.

"There was a small depression by the grave so keep your eyes open for it," I said and led the way through the tangled undergrowth.

We searched for over an hour, crisscrossing the sloping ground but in the end drew a blank.

"I know it was just here," I said, waving my arm in an arc. "It can't just disappear!"

"Well, we haven't found it and now William will really think we were seeing things."

Reluctantly I followed Muriel back to the canoe. The sun continued to shine and we paddled back to the village across a quiet river.

That grave has mystified me for years. I know it was there and my curiosity has never been satisfied. Maybe one of these clear, calm, sunny days, I'll go back and look again.

CHAPTER FIFTEEN

Fort McPherson had changed a lot in the years we
had been away, and Muriel and I decided to walk up to the
north end of the village to look at the site of the old nursing
station. We followed the wooden sidewalk past what had been the
Hudson's Bay Store, now modernized as simply "The Northern." It
was basically the same, although now the front door faced the new
gas pumps instead of opening onto the main road. The riverbank
in front of the Bay manager's house was the place where the village
sages had sat in the summer sun ever since the village had been built.
In the early days they had smoked white clay pipes whose shards
could still be found in the tufts of grass. During our time in Fort
McPherson they would sit on a rickety old bench and smoke their
cigarettes and discuss the topic of the day. They still took a delight in
predicting the weather, looking up at the clouds and remarking on
the direction of the wind before making a prediction, then almost
as insurance—or maybe it was in case someone overheard the prog-
nostication—one or the other would remark, "Funny weather we've
been having lately. It's sure changed since I was a boy. You know we
have never had a year like this before." The others would nod wisely,
showing that they agreed with this profound statement.

The area north of the Bay property was quite changed. Where the
Northern Canada Power Corporation's staff house had stood in the
sixties next to the nursing station only bushes grew now, and to the

north of it where the nursing station, our home for six years, had been, there was only bare ground with a few small trees and brush growing in the yard. At the far end of the property where our warehouse and ice house had been located, a new house had been built for Doris Itsi.

The small Roman Catholic Church that had stood between the nursing station and the home of William and Mary Firth had disappeared, and where their old white clapboard house had been was a large log house that looked out over the Peel River to the west. It had been built in the eighties by the couple's three sons, Ben, Angus and Charlie, and while it had some of the traditional lines of the old houses in the village, it had been designed to accommodate a large family and included indoor plumbing and bathroom facilities. Mary had been a widow by the time it was built, but she lived in it until her death, and it was now the home of her daughter Betty and her family. Unfortunately, we learned that Betty was out of town so we couldn't visit with her.

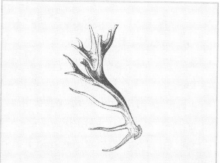

IN THE PAST WHEN WHITE MEN from Outside married Native women, those women automatically lost their Native status and officially became "non-Indian" or "non-status." On the other hand, if a white woman married a Native man, she became a status Indian! Such was the federal government's strange policy.

William Firth's offspring were not registered with the band until the late eighties because William's mother, a Gwich'in, had married John Firth, one of the Hudson's Bay's Scottish factors, so William and his brothers and sisters and their children were not considered Native. When the government policy governing marriage between "status" and "non-status" people was finally changed in April 1985, many people were eligible to regain their Native status.

We were interested to see that most of the Firths and the Blakes still lived at this northern extremity of the village. Agnes Blake and Mary Firth had been very good friends and were possibly related, as were so many people in that small village, and being neighbours, they spent a lot of time together sewing, picking berries or just visiting. They had large families, and as the children had grown and found partners, most of them had built their houses in the same area.

We lingered in front of the vacant space where we had lived, in our minds seeing our old white nursing station still standing there. We had lived and laughed and cried in that building, and we had entertained dozens of people, some willingly, some out of necessity. Dozens of babies had been born there and a number of Gwich'in elders and other community members had died there. We had suffered through inspections and audits and countless other bureaucratic procedures that were, we had to admit, usually necessary.

The clinic room had been very small. There were white-painted cupboards both above and below the countertops on either side of the room, a small sink, a baby scale and an examining table. An adult height and weight scale stood at the end of the examining table. There was a wooden chair just inside the door where patients sat for their consultations, and when an interpreter was present, she had to stand wherever she could. The Gwich'in men never brought an interpreter and we always managed to understand what their problems were, but many of the older women brought an interpreter with them, outlining their problem in Gwich'in to the interpreter who would translate to us. Then I would ask a question in English, and nearly always the patient would answer me directly in English. It was as if some of them needed a little psychological support.

Whenever we had official visitors or friends who had not come for treatment or advice, I was suddenly aware of the antiseptic odour pervading the clinic. Besides prescribing various remedies for our patients, we would also dispense them, pouring liquids for coughs and colds from large Winchester stock bottles into glass medicine

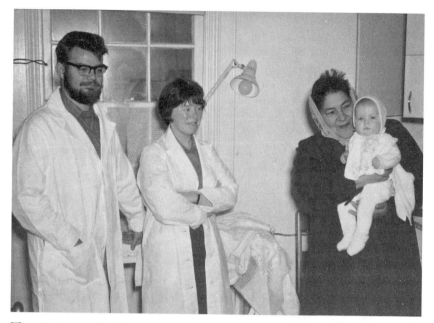

The clinic room had been very small, containing cupboards, a small sink, a baby scale and an examining table.

bottles and using such volatile liquids as oil of cloves for dental patients. With the frequent exposure of these substances, along with various cleansing materials, it was little wonder that the place smelled. Working in this environment on a daily basis made us unaware of it, but after returning from a trip when I had been away for a week or so, I was immediately conscious of it, and I often wondered if this smell was the reason young children were reluctant to come to the clinic. Youngsters, having a very keen sense of smell, would have associated the clinic's odour with the environment where they had been subjected to immunization injections and possibly other indignities.

❅ ❅ ❅

The only family member who visited us from Outside during our six years in Fort McPherson arrived in September 1964. My grandmother, Edith Butler, who was in her late seventies and crippled with rheumatoid arthritis, had written to say that she would have

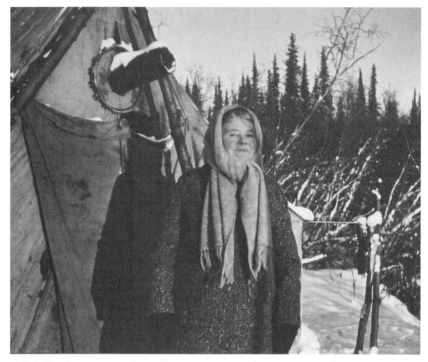

Edith Butler, my grandmother, visits a Gwich'in camp on the Peel River.

liked to visit us in Fort McPherson if it hadn't been so far away. She
had come from Britain to visit her son, my uncle, in southern Ontario, and while she was there, we had written to tell her that Muriel
was expecting our first child that December. Her reply hinted that a
visit to us would be so nice, but after consulting a map, she had decided that, as we were so far away, it would be too expensive to come.
The idea of travelling thousands of kilometres to Fort McPherson
from Britain must have seemed like going to the ends of the earth.
But my grandparents had been a great influence on my early years
when I had lived with them, and I had always felt very close to my
grandmother especially, (my grandfather had died many years earlier). In fact, Muriel insisted that I had only married her because she
reminded me of my grandmother! So now we discussed the situation and decided that, if we were to send a plane ticket for her to
fly from Ontario to Inuvik, she would not be able to refuse. So we

bought the ticket, and when she received it, she was so overcome that she made immediate arrangements to come North.

She flew from Toronto to Edmonton where our friends there met her and cared for her until the plane to carry her to Inuvik was due. I had arranged to go to Inuvik to meet her, but at the last moment an emergency prevented me from leaving Fort McPherson on that day. What was a genteel, elderly English lady, suffering from crippling rheumatoid arthritis, going to do when she arrived in the Far North and was more or less dumped at the airport? Fortunately, we had met Mr. and Mrs. Mockford, Inuvik's Anglican minister and his wife, when they had visited Fort McPherson. We did not really know them and we did not belong to the Anglican Church, but they were English and we hoped that they would understand the predicament we were in. One long explanatory phone call quickly settled everything, and Mrs. Mockford said that she would be happy to meet my grandmother and take her to their home.

"But how will I recognize her?" she asked

"She will look like a little old English lady," I replied.

All went well and by early afternoon on September 14 my grandmother was sipping tea in the manse. When she had left Toronto the previous day the temperature was in the mid-thirties (C) and when she arrived in Inuvik there had been a fresh fall of snow and the temperature was minus six!

Meanwhile, I had been called to an accident at one of the Imperial Oil exploration camps about an hour's ride from Fort McPherson. I crossed the Peel River in a scow, and just as I was wondering how the company dispatcher and I were to travel to the camp, I was suddenly confronted by a large tracked vehicle called a Nodwell. I clambered into the machine, the driver started up the noisy engine and we lurched off over the tundra and were soon at the camp. My patient had fallen and injured his back and was in a lot of pain, and it didn't take a long examination to see that he would have to be evacuated to hospital. We strapped him to a spinal board, I gave him an injection to ease his pain, and then we carefully lifted him into the Nodwell. After our lurching ride up to the camp, I was worried about how my patient would manage. The driver drove very slowly, but even so we all were thrown about in the Nodwell's cab.

Eventually we arrived at the river and with the help of Imperial Oil Company workers we were able to get the patient over to the east side of the river where the plane that had been called by the camp expediter was waiting. I sent a message to Muriel that I was escorting the patient to hospital. In Inuvik the patient was admitted to hospital and it was quickly decided that he should be sent out to Edmonton on the next Mainliner, as the Pacific Western Airlines plane was called.

This one man's unfortunate accident enabled me to greet my grandmother in Inuvik, albeit a few hours later than planned, and I was overjoyed to see her. Mrs. Mockford asked if my grandmother could stay the night with them, and as it was too late to fly to Fort McPherson that day, I was quite happy with this arrangement. When I went off to the hospital staff quarters, I left the two women knitting, drinking tea and discussing the affairs of Britain.

By noon the next day we were in Fort McPherson, and Muriel, six months pregnant, was there to greet my grandmother. Although we had to continue our everyday schedules, Grandma was happy to sit in an easy chair in our living room and keep busy with her knitting needles. Rachel Stuart brought her tea and cookies and they had a somewhat stilted conversation until we were able to spend time with her. When the weather was nice we would go for walks, laughing as the sticky mud tried to suck off Grandma's boots.

When some of the older ladies in the village, especially those who had experienced the difficulties and rigours of travelling, had heard that my aged grandmother was going to visit from far away, they were delighted. Now they came to visit and drink tea. I had warned my grandmother that the women didn't talk much so she just sat and knitted and talked a little. She didn't seem to mind sitting quietly there during the silent periods, but I don't think she understood very much of the conversation when they did speak.

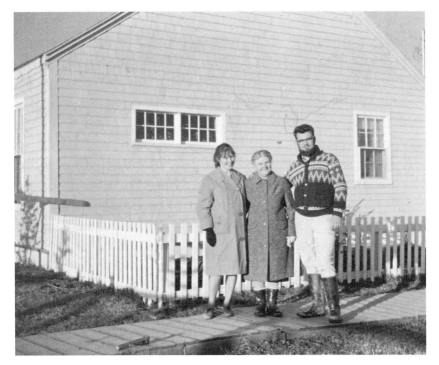

Edith Butler heads out for a walk outside the nursing station.

However, her visitors were fascinated that my grandmother's bent and twisted arthritic fingers could convert a ball of wool into a recognizable piece of baby clothing.

We were not too sure how long my grandmother's visit was to last, and in the end I had to ask her so I could think about arranging transportation. We knew, however, that we would not be going anywhere for a while because shortly after her arrival all the planes went south for their overhaul and the annual changeover from pontoons to skis.

"I'd really like to stay until after the baby is born," Grandma said.

This put us into a quandary because, when Muriel went to Inuvik for delivery, I wanted to be with her, and I could hardly leave my grandmother in the nursing station alone. Fortunately she understood our predicament and offered a compromise. "I'll go after I have had a dog team ride!"

A few days later a call from the head office advised me that I was to attend a conference in Yellowknife on November 12, and we realized that this would resolve our problems. As Yellowknife was well on the way to Edmonton, I could escort my grandmother that far and she could continue to Edmonton and Toronto under the care of various friends and relatives. By the end of October there was enough snow on the ground for a dog team to pull a toboggan without any problems, and William Firth reported that a trail had already been made down the river where someone fishing for losh had set up a tent. As soon as I had the team hitched up and ready to go, Muriel sat in the toboggan with her back against the lazyback and then my grandmother was eased into the toboggan so Muriel was supporting her frail frame. They were both wrapped in a heavy sleeping bag, the collar on Grandma's English woolen coat was pulled up and a scarf was wrapped around her head. I couldn't help thinking that if the toboggan tipped, I would have a very pregnant wife and an elderly crippled lady lying in the snow, and I rode the brake as much as possible to keep the eager dogs in check, but once we were off the road and onto the bush trail we all settled down. We headed into a cold north wind, but Grandma didn't complain and hung on tight to the carriole. When we arrived at the tent, no one was there so we had a look around, took some photographs and headed back. When the dogs entered the yard, William appeared and took them over while I untangled Muriel and Grandma from the sleeping bag and led them inside. As Grandma took off her coat, Muriel remarked that it looked as though she had frostbitten her neck, and sure enough a section of Grandma's neck that had not been covered by her scarf was very red. But she didn't mind at all, and for days afterward whenever anyone came by, she would show them her neck and say, "I got my neck frostbitten when I was out on a dog team trip with Keith!" Talk about war wounds!

The time came when farewells had to be said, and leaving a very pregnant Muriel behind, Grandma and I went off to Yellowknife. We'd had a wonderful visit, and I knew that the elders in the

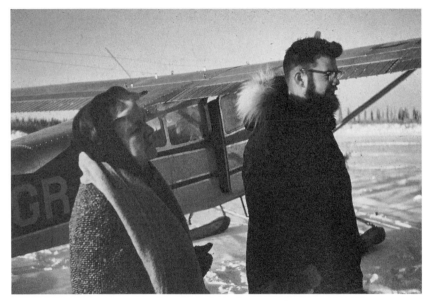

Parting is such sweet sorrow: Edith Butler leaves Fort McPherson with her grandson, bound for Yellowknife.

village had been quite impressed by my travelling grandmother!

❊　❊　❊

Resuming our memory walk along the bank of the Peel River, Muriel and I passed a hedge that was already losing its leaves. We stopped, looked at each other and began to laugh. Long ago Mary Firth had told us that, whenever she took our son, Stephen, down to her house, he had stopped to urinate on this same bush, and after it happened a few times she started calling it "Stephen's pee tree!" And here it was all these years later still struggling to survive.

When we arrived at the place where the old dock had been and where supplies had been unloaded from the barges, only a few rotting logs remained to mark the spot, and a sea of willows and small spruce that had grown up on the sand bar below the village. The Peel River, which averages about six knots as it sweeps past this point, plays cat and mouse with the village of Fort McPherson, which stands on a high bank of shale on its eastern side. In the mid-forties the river flowed close to this bank, and supply boats such as the

Distributor had been able to off-load right below the village. But the Peel flows over four hundred kilometres from its source in the Ogilvie Mountains to the point where it meets the Mackenzie in the Delta, and it picks up and carries tonnes of sediment downriver, so in spite of some dredging operations, over the years a large sand-bar built up below the village. By the mid-sixties the river itself was nearly a hundred metres from the bank, and the barges had to be off-loaded about a kilometre and a half to the north where the water was deep enough close to the riverbank and the supplies could be placed in a secure and dry area.

When the Gwich'in of old had come to the village in the spring-time to replenish their supplies of staple items, it had been customary to greet the wood-burning steamboat bringing supplies and visitors to the fort with volleys of rifle fire. The same thing occurred when the boat pulled away from shore after discharging its load of goods and taking on board the year's accumulation of furs. The Gwich'in then returned to their camps with all the necessary things that were now required for bush living: ammunition, fishing hooks and nets, tea, sugar, hardware such as stoves and tin chimneys, axes and files.

When we arrived in Fort McPherson in September 1963, one of the first chores we had to undertake was ordering the supplies for the following year. They would be delivered to the Northern Transportation Company's depot at Waterways, Alberta, on the Athabasca River. Here goods destined for the North were assembled at the docks as they were received by truck and train from everywhere across the whole country, if not the world. Then as soon as spring breakup began on the Athabasca, a ship equipped with sonar would start to follow the outgoing ice in order to locate new sandbars and shoals, and markers would be set along the shore as guides to the deeper channels. These markers were then drawn onto a narrow, de-tailed map of the river, which was mounted onto rollers in the pilot houses of the river boats. When all was ready, tugboats such as the thirty-metre-long *Pelican Rapids* would set off down the Macken-zie pushing a flotilla of loaded rafts or barges. (These barges were also known locally as "tows," although they were actually pushed in front of the tugs.) As they proceeded down the river, the helmsman unrolled the map to avoid the new sandbars and shoals. When the *Pelican Rapids* had negotiated its way north up the Athabasca, across Great Slave Lake and on up the Mackenzie to the Mouth of the Peel, the crew would tie up the rafts that were destined for farther north and take three or four of the rafts up the narrower and winding Peel River.

Having been warned that if our supply order did not reach head office in time for them to approve and process it, we might end up on short rations the following year, Muriel took on this responsibility. However, ordering such large quantities of food was quite foreign to both of us. We were in our early twenties and newly married; the only experience that we had of shopping was visiting the local IGA in Edmonton to get a weeks' supply of groceries. But necessity works wonders, and our order for groceries and all the medical and cleaning supplies needed for the nursing station was sent in on time, and then we waited expectantly for the barge to come in with crates and boxes clearly labelled "Health and Welfare." When these were located amid the pile of crates on the dock and brought to the station, with the help of William Firth we packed everything into our heated warehouse. William had being doing this ever since the station had been built so he knew the routine very well and was a great help to us. He explained that the crates of "fresh" eggs we had received would last longer if we put them in the cooler part of the warehouse, and he told us he would come and turn the cases every week. Later in the year after opening a few eggs that had a distinctly greenish colour and smelled slightly sulphuric, we learned to break the egg into a cup first, and if it still resembled what we remembered about eggs, we would use it.

During that first winter we were very happy to discover that from time to time the staff at the Inuvik General Hospital would send fresh produce to us by plane if they had a surplus. It was so nice to open a box and find fresh lettuce, even though it had sometimes been touched by frost—having sat at the airstrip for a few minutes in minus forty degree weather—but it had to be pretty bad before we rejected it. Sometimes we received some really fresh eggs, maybe only a week old, and we delighted in having just one each for breakfast so they would last us for awhile.

In the later years that we served at Fort McPherson someone down south had an epiphany and realized that the shelves of the Hudson's Bay Company were full of the tins of food that we were also ordering and storing, and as a result we were directed to get all of our future supplies through the Bay. We were given a generous financial limit for spending on food and other supplies (we were classified as two single people for staffing needs), and we were also allowed to buy the extra food and supplies that were needed when we had in-patients at the nursing station. As most of the Bay managers had come from England or Scotland themselves, they were very cooperative and ordered items that they knew we liked, and when the barges arrived at the dock in the summer time we would go down to watch, feeling quite pleased that we no longer had to worry about food supplies. As soon as our medical supplies were found and William sent them up to the nursing station, we could relax.

On one of these days when we were standing idly by watching the storekeepers, the Indian agent, the school janitor and the RCMP all busily rounding up their precious goods, Alex Forman, one of the free traders, called over to me to ask if I had a driver's licence, and if I had, how about driving one of his trucks for him because nobody else who was available had a licence. I thought that maybe he was asking because the RCMP were at the dock, but they were all working and I doubted they would have issued a ticket even if they had one to issue. I had never driven a big commercial truck before and didn't think my licence would cover me, but as it was Saturday, I thought, *Why not?* Muriel told me to go ahead if I wanted to. Alex explained that when the truck was loaded it wouldn't go above first gear, so I had no need to worry, but he warned me to take it easy on the return trip because the road was muddy and greasy. "I've got enough boys to load and unload so all you have to do is drive and stay on the road."

I worked until about two in the morning making trip after trip and quite enjoyed myself. As it stayed light all night at that time of the year with the sun setting at about midnight and rising again an hour later, I could quite honestly say that I had driven from sunset to sunrise. To add to my pleasure, after we finished the job, Alex thrust fifty dollars into my hand. "Thanks," he said. "That worked out quite well." And I went away thinking that I now had something unique to add to my resume!

I had also been taught how to drive a small Caterpillar tractor by, of all people, the Hudson's Bay store manager in Arctic Red River. I had gone down to the Mackenzie River with him when he was hauling the dock out of the water prior to freezeup, and when he finished, he asked me if I would like to try driving it. Always eager for fresh experiences, I jumped at the opportunity and after a quick lesson I ran the machine up and down the shore enjoying myself like a kid with a new toy.

CHAPTER SIXTEEN

O N MANY POSTCARDS AND PHOTOGRAPHS, AND even on some souvenirs, there is a photograph of Fort McPherson's old St. Matthews Mission taken from the south. On the left-hand side there is a pine tree, and it is growing in the corner of the graveyard just behind the Mission House. There is nothing fantastic about this tree except that over the years it has changed along with everything else, and now when we walked along the riverbank, we noticed that the tree was bigger, more noticeable. And this was how all of Fort McPherson appeared to us as we looked around forty years later. Things were the same, but somehow more noticeable. The buildings no longer had the old character; instead they had a new character that reflected the changes and improvements in the Gwich'in community in general.

But the graveyard still reflected the history of the Gwich'in because you cannot walk around in it without feeling the memories that it holds. As Muriel and I toured it, we were disheartened to see the many graves of our old friends. Many of the simple wooden crosses marking them were falling into disrepair and some had gone altogether, leaving just a grassy mound to show that a body was lying in the permafrost. Granite headstones marked the newer graves because the coming of the Dempster Highway had made it possible for people to have them shipped in from the south and many of them now had photographs pasted on them as well.

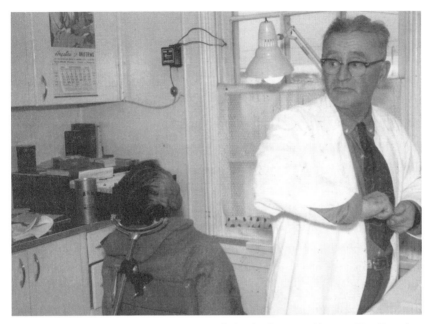

A rare occurrence: William Vittrekwa (who had no teeth) visits Dr. Dowler, DDS, on a rare dental clinic in Fort McPherson.

For me one grave stood out from the rest. It was that of William Vittrekwa. Where William Firth had been almost like a father to me and guided me through the community, William Vittrekwa had been my bush teacher, and a very practical teacher he had been. He was friends with William and Mary Firth and we always had to be careful when referring to "William and Mary" as both Williams were married to Marys, and both were in the same age bracket. But while William Firth had been educated and worked for the Bay, William Vittrekwa had only a rudimentary formal education. Instead, his school had been the land itself, and he knew the habits and locality of all the animals. He put nets into the Peel River for his annual supply of fish, but I always had the idea that the mountains were the place that he loved most. He and Mary spent long months there every year hunting caribou, drying it and making "itsoo." William would also hunt moose all alone and most of the time he was quite successful.

Neither Muriel or I ever had to treat him for illness, and the only time that he came to the clinic was to see a dentist, Dr. Dowler, who was visiting the settlement for a short time. I wasn't sure why William came to see him because I don't think he had a tooth in his head, and when he laughed, which he did quite often, his shiny gums would be evident. If he'd had teeth, he would have had a malocclusion where the lower jaw is thrust forward making the bottom teeth come up over the top set.

William Vittrekwa, like William Firth, seemed to sense when it was coffee time, especially when a new batch of cinnamon rolls or muffins had come out of the oven, and it was almost more than I could do to keep a straight face to see both Williams munching away on these goodies without a tooth between them. He was one of the few Gwich'in people who came to the kitchen door and walked in rather than going formally to the clinic door. If the clinic was quiet he would stay and chat, and Muriel and I were happy to listen to his stories. His English was passable and we could understand most of what he was telling us because he used facial expressions and waved his arms to indicate large mountains, and his hands were transformed into dog teams or running caribou or a hunter shooting with a rifle. He always had some grandiose scheme that involved us spending money on planes or helicopters while he showed us some part of the country. He would sit in the kitchen chair, remove his salt-and-pepper floppy tweed cap to reveal a mass of trimmed straight grey hair, and after a sip or two of coffee, he would tell us where he had been and that we really should go ourselves.

In the bitterly cold weather he had been known to go hunting, staying out for days, and besides his rifle and shells he would have only some dried meat and tea and carry a grey blanket. At night when he made camp, a camp that would have frozen me, he would make tea on a fire, then when the embers burned down he would straddle the fire with the blanket pulled around his shoulders and stay there until he was rested up. This was when he was seventy years old! I could not imagine him being worried by anything in the bush, and yet he told me that one day when he had been hunting caribou in the fall, he had been coming down the mountain following a narrow creek that was full of large boulders when he saw a huge grizzly bear coming up the creek toward him. He immediately crouched behind a boulder and silently checked his rifle. He did not want to open the breech to see how many shells he had in it because he did not want to make any noise. The grizzly was so close, he said, that if it had smelled him or decided to charge him, he would not have had time to shoot, and he wasn't sure if he had enough shells to shoot anyway. He said that he barely breathed and his heart was pounding with fright, and when the bear was passing, he couldn't see it from where he was hiding behind the rock and he thought that the bear might just come up behind him. He stayed there for "a long time"— I thought this might have been a minute or two because I knew what he meant. It was that moment when time stands still. When he heard a rock fall some distance above him, he strained his neck and looked slowly up the creek and with relief saw the rear end of the bear continuing up the creek. He said he still waited for some time before getting up and moving quietly down the creek. It was then that he checked his rifle and saw that he only had three shells in the breech.

One day he came to tell us that he had recently come down from Vittrekwa Creek, and along the way he had seen moose sign at the entrance to the creek. Now he was heading back to see if he could find that old moose. "I'm just going one day, maybe two. You should come. No one left in town anyway. Bring camera." The Gwich'in usually hunted moose early in the fall when they were fat from a summer of grazing, as the fat was prized for cooking, and for mixing with berries and pulverized dried meat to make a form of pemmican, which the Gwich'in called "itsoo."

I felt that it was a great honour to be asked to go hunting with this old man and I wanted to jump at the chance, but if I went, even for "one day, maybe two," Muriel would be alone in the nursing station again and one of our patients was expecting her baby at any time.

"I don't mind if you go." Muriel had read my thoughts. "I would like to go, too, but with that baby due, I had better stay around. And anyway, moose hunting doesn't really appeal to me."

When William had said there was no one left in town, it was a bit of an exaggeration because there must have been almost half the population still in the settlement, with the children staying in Fleming Hall, young mothers and some of the old people, plus the white people and those who worked at the Bay and the NCPC. But to convince myself and Muriel, I repeated out loud, "It is *very* quiet in the clinic at present!"

Early the next morning old William and I were heading up the Peel River toward Vittrekwa Creek behind our dog teams. The trip was about forty kilometres and William thought that we should be there before dark. He had a team of large, exceptionally hairy dogs, which, because they were in almost constant use, were well trained and obedient. He never shouted at them and always looked after them well. If one of his dogs got twisted in the harness, he would stop the team and make sure that the dog's leg was not injured.

Later William was with me when we went by dogsled to Dawson City, and a few kilometres from our destination one of his dogs was pulling so hard that its lungs hemorrhaged and it died. Tough old William was as close to tears as he had ever been when he was telling me about it. I was surprised at this old hunter who had killed hundreds of animals for food and fur, but he evidently had a special relationship with his faithful dogs.

Some people, mostly the younger generation, treated their dogs cruelly and the dogs would cower when they approached. I once saw a young man get so mad at his dogs that he ran to the bush, broke a large branch off a tree and proceeded to beat the animal with it, breaking its leg. It was then no good as a sled dog and had to be put down. Fortunately, there were not too many dog owners like that. My own patience has been tried many times by some of the dogs I have used, and once when I wanted the lead dog to turn off the main trail and onto another infrequently used trail, the dog would not turn,

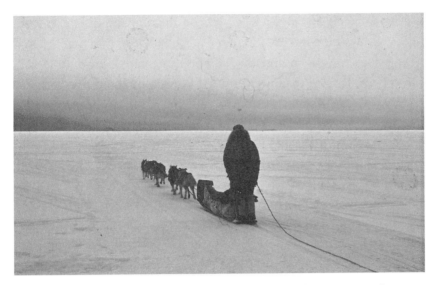

The cold road home: my own patience has been tried many times by some of the dogs.

so I got off the toboggan and pulled him over to the trail I wanted him to take. Then standing on the toboggan, I urged the dogs on. To my absolute frustration the dog went forward a few paces and then swung back onto the other trail again. I called for him to turn to the right, but he wouldn't budge, so I went forward again and pulled him through the snow onto the correct trail again and tried to set off. He did the same thing again. This time I stormed up to him and gave him a swift kick with my mukluk. Then I was really mad because it appeared that I had broken my toe when I kicked him. I grabbed his collar and shouted in his ear, "You go on *this* trail!" and at the same moment I had a moment of madness when I really felt like biting his ear! When I stopped long enough to assess my feelings, I laughed in spite of my injured toe, and then limping, I dragged the reluctant lead dog down the trail a short way and tried again. I think the dog now felt sorry for me and this time to humour me went obediently in the direction I wanted him to go.

William and I travelled up the river, my dogs following close on his heels. He didn't speak to his dogs at all but rode along quietly. I usually spoke to my dogs when I was on the trail and their ears were nearly always tuned to my direction, but I had been told that I talked to the dogs too much and this stopped them from travelling well. On this trip I tried to contain myself. It took us about five hours to reach Vittrekwa Creek, although William never knew the time of day and never wore a watch. His only comment when I asked him about time was something to the effect that his stomach told him when it was time to eat and when it was dark he went to bed. He located a place where we were going to camp and told me to flatten an area of snow where he could set the canvas tent. I was relieved to see that he did not expect me to squat over some hot coals overnight.

It was an education to see him work. He used a fraction of the axe strokes that I used to cut down a tree, and by the time the tent was set, the evergreen branches put down on the floor and the wood stove in place, I was feeling very inferior to this "old" man. But although he knew that he was far superior to me in the bush, he never said anything to put me down. My sense of inferiority came from knowing that I could not survive without him.

He was a born actor and loved to perform for the benefit of anyone around, even if it was an audience of one. If he saw a camera, his casual persona would change and he would pose as he thought a mighty hunter would pose, and when I took some home movies of him, his actions were always exaggerated, making me laugh. Sometimes I would hold the camera without having it switched on and try to capture his actions when he was not expecting it. I guess that over the years he had guided too many people who had cameras!

It was too late to do any hunting that day so we made a big fire in a pile of driftwood at the edge of the creek, cooked the dog feed and then our own supper. When everybody and everything had been fed, we went into the tent, rolled out our sleeping bags and sat back with cups of tea as we waited for the sleeping bags to warm up in the heat from the wood stove. It was quiet in the tent as old William sat there nursing his tea and staring at the glowing stove. Like the other Gwich'in men I had travelled with, he never talked unless there was something of note to discuss. He did not need to chatter or even listen to the radio. Instead, he listened to the wind and the other noises outside, interpreting each sound. By the look in his eyes I suspected that he was thinking about the past as many older people do, and later he told me a few stories of his earlier life and about his father. He never mentioned his mother and I wondered if this reflected the status of women in those days or perhaps just indicated she had died while he was still a youngster.

He said that when he was a young boy, he had been trained to go long distances and that he was only allowed to drink the amount of water that could be held in a squirrel skull. I could not get a definitive answer from him about how often he was allowed this amount of water, but he said it was so he could run over the mountains without feeling thirsty. I wondered if it was part of a coming of age puberty rite for boys, but unfortunately I did not know how to phrase my questions so he could understand.

Lying there in the tent gave me the opportunity to reflect on the day, to think of home and compare it with the environment I was now in. I had lots of questions because my knowledge of the Gwich'in life and history was so limited, so whenever I saw William stir for a moment to put a log on the fire, I knew his thoughts had been interrupted, and I would ask, "Why is this like this?" or "What do you do when . . .?" He would answer my questions in his own peculiar brand of English, which I had found hard to understand at first, though as time went on I found that the more I listened the clearer the answers became. I even found myself speaking in the same manner.

As I snuggled down in my sleeping bag, William told me that my Woods Three Star sleeping bag was much too heavy and would take up too much room in the toboggan, and he showed me his summer weight kapok bag that must have weighed all of one and a half kilograms. "This one, he's good. No use to have that big blanket." But that bag was something I would never relinquish because if I could sleep well through the coldest nights, I knew that I could survive the days that followed. I awoke sometime in the middle of the night and could feel the cold on my face, and though the stove had long gone out I was quite warm. It was comforting to hear William's steady breathing and to smell the pungent aroma of the pine boughs beneath me. I pulled my toque down over my ears and went back to sleep.

I heard William stirring early in the morning when it was still dark. He was fumbling around near the stove and then I was dazzled as he struck a match and touched it to some feather sticks in the stove. I listened to the sound of the crackling fire and soon the smell of woodsmoke drifted through the tent. When I heard the tea pail bubbling, I sat up. We ate bacon and porridge for breakfast, which was more my traditional breakfast than William's, except that he poured the bacon fat over his porridge oats, telling me that the fat would keep him warm. I preferred sugar.

After several cups of sweet, strong tea, we donned our parkas and went out into the half light and put on our snowshoes. As we walked up Vittrekwa Creek, the dogs howled their disappointment at being left behind, but after we had gone around the first bend the deep snow and the creek banks swallowed up every sound and all we could hear was the rhythmic swish, swish of our snowshoes on the granular snow.

The mouth of Vittrekwa Creek was almost plugged with willow islands, and it is in places like this that moose come in winter because the willows provide them with both food and protection from the wind. When the weather was very bad and the winds bitterly cold, moose were known to congregate in large numbers on islands like this, and I had once been fortunate enough to fly with the game warden to the head of the Arctic Red River when he was doing a game count. The temperature was minus forty, and as we flew over, we saw dozens of moose gathered together in quite close proximity. Our pilot, Freddy Carmichael, was unable to land his small plane, but I was quite satisfied to watch almost with disbelief as we saw all those moose within a sheltered draw of the river.

William was confident that the tracks that he had seen earlier would lead him to a moose, but it was only after we had been out for an hour that he came across the old prints. He said that the moose would still be in the area and probably wouldn't move around much because of the cold unless, of course, he was disturbed. We started following the tracks and it was plain that the moose was browsing in the area because his tracks crossed over each other. William said they were about two days old, but they all looked the same to me. We walked all day and I was tired and hot in my heavy parka and had given up all hope of seeing a moose, but William went doggedly on so I said nothing. I would have been quite happy to turn around and go back to camp, but my pride would not let me give in when this seventy-year-old man showed no inclination to quit.

We followed the tracks along a small tributary creek and then snowshoed up the steep bank where the moose had gone. Snowshoes are hard enough to walk on when you are on a flat surface and you have not had much practice, and now I found that it was equally difficult to climb up a steep bank with them on. William did not even slow his pace as he climbed the bank and he was breaking trail! I went forward two steps and then slid back. I got my snowshoes crossed between two willows, and then while trying to extricate myself, I dropped my gun in the snow and the breech and barrel were filled with snow. I was lathered in sweat and annoyed at my ineptitude.

It was not my snowshoes' fault. They had been custom-made by a real Gwich'in artisan, Ronnie Pascal, for my height and weight in the traditional Gwich'in style with hand-carved wood, curved rounded fronts and tapered backs with finely woven babiche in the front and back and coarser babiche under the soles of the feet. The wood had been stained red with a clay that was obtained on a hidden hillside that I was told had a spiritual significance. And when the clay was taken, a gift of some value to the taker had to be left in return—maybe tobacco, tea or sugar or something similar.

Meanwhile, William was almost out of sight and still after his moose. I gave up trying to keep up with him and inched my way forward, pulling myself up by hanging onto trees wherever I could, knowing that as far as I was concerned the moose was quite safe. I was just pushing myself out of another snowbank when I saw William coming toward me.

"More better you go back. That moose he gone up over. I go maybe see him." And with that he turned and went back along his trail. He hadn't questioned why I was going so slowly. He had just stated a simple fact. I should go back, he would go on. It made perfect sense and I was relieved. Several hours later I was back in camp after following our snowshoe trail. I lit the stove, made tea and changed my clothes then lay back thankfully on my sleeping bag. After dozing for a while I had a snack, and as the light faded I cooked dog feed and fed both teams.

William returned long after dark. He was very tired and did not say very much until after drinking tea and eating some of the meat I had fried. He then sat back and told me that the moose must have heard the dogs early in the morning and after reaching the top of the creek it had taken off quickly. I did wonder if the moose had heard me thrashing around in the creek and William was being too polite to say so and instead blamed the dogs. He had trailed the moose a long way before turning back, and I think he was disappointed for me as much as for himself.

I had cooked some rice to go with the meat and just as I was wondering what to do with what was left, William asked, "You like berries?"

"I sure do. You got some?"

He didn't answer but fished around in his pack and pulled out a small canvas bag filled with some dried red berries. "Here." He offered me the bag. "Some whitemen, he doesn't like these too much."

"What are they? Cranberries?"

"Maybe they are. I don't know the name in English."

I decided to try them and poured several spoons full into my rice, mixed them together, then put a spoonful into my mouth. They were sharp tasting but not unpleasant, so I chewed the mouthful, and then feeling that I had broken a tooth, I pulled the bits out of my mouth and saw that each of these berries had two tiny rock-hard seeds in them.

"You like 'em?" William asked as he watched me.

"They taste fine but they've got a lot of seeds in them." I spat out some of the seeds.

"Aha. That's what they're like." William ate some berries himself and swallowed, and it occurred to me that this must be one of the benefits of having no teeth.

It took me a long time to finish my portion, along with much crunching and spitting which expressed my feeling admirably.

We broke camp early the next morning and headed for home. William was quite philosophical and said, "Maybe I get that moose in the spring. He more fat then!"

He would get a moose, of that I was certain. It was what he did, it was his life. He had showed me that age did not mean anything in the bush, and though he looked old and hadn't got a tooth in his head, he could chew a mouthful of seedy berries without a problem and run circles around me anytime. And he knew it, too. So it was that I realized that you are as old as you feel. The Gwich'in worked hard all their lives so they were able to do things without any strain that would be physically difficult for southerners to accomplish at all. In those days I never did hear of a Gwich'in person who had to enroll in an exercise program to keep fit. They were the role models for the saying: "If you use it, you won't lose it!"

Although there is always sadness when you see the graves of so many loved ones, those graves can also be inspiring when you think of the lives of some of the people who lie there, each one with a story, some sad, some glad, some of incredible hardship. But there was one story connected to the mission church that had a happier ending, one that did not end in the graveyard. In 1909 Isaac Stringer, the bishop for the Mackenzie area, had set out in late summer for the Rat River then over the mountains to Fort Yukon and Dawson City. Stringer was accompanied by another missionary named Charles Johnson, who was leaving the North to be with his family, and a third missionary named Fry was to accompany them partway. As well, they had hired two Gwich'in guides from Fort McPherson, Enoch Moses and Joe Vittrekwa.

Hudson's Bay factor John Firth and his wife saw them off down the Peel River. They reached the Husky Channel, turned up the Rat River and worked hard against the current until they reached the rapids. It was here that Enoch Moses feigned sickness and announced that he couldn't go on, and Stringer and Vittrekwa took him back to Fort McPherson where Moses soon recovered. (Bishop Springer found out later that Moses had done this to previous parties.) In Fort McPherson Stringer hired another man to guide them but they had now lost a week's travel time.

On the second attempt they had a very hard time tracking up the Rat River but finally reached the Divide. Here, as previously arranged, the two Gwich'in men and Fry turned back as the current of the rivers, now all running west, would be with the travellers. The weather had now turned cold, and because of the week's delay, they were already short of rations and game was scarce in the area, but the two men set off together just as it started to snow. As the weather got colder, they had to break the ice forming on the river in order to move their small canvas canoe. They were hoping to reach the Porcupine River, which might still be open, but after several days of very slow progress, they decided to take a shortcut across the mountains to Lapierre House then go back to Fort McPherson, a distance of about 160 kilometres. They cached their canoe and set out with small packs. Neither of them had snowshoes and the snow made walking very difficult.

With only a small map and a compass to guide them, they could not find Lapierre House and decided to go instead right across the mountains directly to Fort McPherson. They crossed and recrossed partially frozen creeks, which left them wet and cold, and then fog surrounded them so that they found it difficult to negotiate the mountain precipices. There was no game and they were almost out of food. There were no trees for shelter as they crossed the tundra and no wood to make a fire, so they camped out in the open wrapped in their wet blankets and clothes. After days of this suffering they decided to go down into the valley where they might find shelter and wood for a fire as well as material to make snowshoes, something neither had made before. Over the next few days they camped in the open while they constructed makeshift snowshoes.

By now they were slowly starving to death and found it hard to stay awake, so they took turns resting, one always keeping watch, as they were frightened that, if they both fell asleep, they might not wake up. Then Stringer remembered a tale of a starving Indian who had survived by eating boiled beaver skins, so in desperation the men now boiled their Eskimo mukluks, providing them with some nourishment. After four days of this diet, they came to a large river, which they gathered was the Peel after they cut a hole in the ice to see which way it was flowing. They followed the river until they came to an old camp and at the same time saw smoke from a nearby Indian camp, which turned out to be that of William Vittrekwa and two other men. The Gwich'in were surprised and shocked to see the two missionaries and didn't recognize them at first as each man had lost over twenty-two kilograms in the past month. They fed the two starving men and then took them down the river to Fort McPherson by dogsled where they were received with shock and then thankfulness.

It was just two years later in 1911 that a real tragedy occurred when four Royal North West Mounted Policemen perished after trying to travel to Dawson City from Fort McPherson without a Gwich'in guide. They, like Isaac Stringer, turned back, but they then died along the way, Inspector Fitzgerald, the leader of the patrol succumbing last, just thirty-two kilometres from Fort McPherson.

Ken Snyder, who organized the Dawson City Welcome Committee for the 1970 Centennial Dawson Patrol from Fort McPherson, described the RNWMP police patrols by saying:

The patrol system was a feature of police history by which small detachments of men would make long trips in the winter season in order to keep the remotest part in touch with civilization. They carried mail to points that would otherwise be completely isolated and this gave some relief to the men besides providing some oversight of these wilderness regions. These patrols were frequent through the years and they all exemplified courage and endurance of a very high type. Deeds took place on these wilderness patrols that, if done in other fields, would have won highly prized decorations. On patrol, they were the regular order of the day, unseen by human eyes, unnoticed by the public, and when the men who wrought these deeds reported them, it was in a self-deprecating way that only those who understood guessed at the tale of heroism that lay behind their simple statement.

When the RNWMP patrol left Fort McPherson on December 21, 1910, the temperature was minus twenty-nine (C) and there was a north wind behind them. A day or two later it snowed. On Christmas Day they reached a cache of fish that had been taken there for them previously by one of the constables. From this point on they experienced heavy going in deep snow, and Fitzgerald wrote in his diary that they were breaking trail through nine metres of snow. They then made their wisest move of the whole trip by hiring a Gwich'in man and his dog team to help them cross a 128-kilometre portage, which took them to an altitude of over three hundred metres. On December 30 it was minus forty-six (C) and the snow in the creeks along which they were travelling was very deep.

On January 1 Fitzgerald paid off the guide because Carter, a special constable with the patrol, said that he knew the way. After this they made only sixteen to twenty kilometres a day as the thick bush, heavy snow and cold temperatures slowed them right down. On January 8 Fitzgerald recorded a low of minus fifty-three (C), although by January 10 the temperature had risen again to minus twenty-five (C). One week later, after they had journeyed up one creek after another looking for a portage, Fitzgerald realized that Carter did not know the route, and he wrote in his journal, "Carter is completely lost and does not know where to go." He decided to turn the patrol around and return to Fort McPherson. But their rations were now very low and it became necessary to kill some of the dogs to feed their remaining animals, but when the other dogs refused to eat the meat, the men had to feed them dryfish and eat the dog meat themselves.

Misty weather on the high ground and overflow on the creeks made for a miserable few days, and this was followed by days of high winds and glare ice. The temperature now dipped again to minus fifty-three (C). They found themselves walking in overflow on the creeks and some of the men suffered from frostbite. Taylor and Carter fell into an open stretch of water up to their waists so camp had to be made quickly to dry them out. Day by day their progress slowed as the trail they had made on their outward journey had been obliterated by fresh snowfalls and the number of dogs was dwindling as they shot and ate them. By January 30 they were all feeling ill and the skin was peeling from their faces. Fitzgerald thought it was from eating the dogs' livers. By February 5 they were down to five dogs and the temperature was minus forty-four (C) when Fitzgerald fell through the ice and they had to stop and make a fire for him.

While the patrol was struggling on the trail back to Fort McPherson, the Gwich'in guide who had assisted the party over the long portage arrived in Dawson City and reported where he had last seen the party. But the alarm was not raised until another party of Gwich'in arrived in Dawson from the Hart River and said they had seen nothing of the patrol. On February 28 a relief party headed by Corporal William John Duncan Dempster left Dawson with three dog teams. On March 12 Dempster's party came across an old trail on the Little Wind River and realized that Fitzgerald must have turned back. Later they found some old camps, and by the cans and a piece of a flour sack with RNWMP stamped on it, they knew they were on the right track. When they came across an old cabin where a toboggan and seven sets of dog harness were cached and then found the paws of a dog and a shoulder blade from which they could see the meat had been cooked and eaten, Dempster knew that the patrol they were looking for was in dire straits.

On March 21 Dempster's party found an open camp in which there were two bodies, those of Constable Kinney and Constable Taylor. Taylor still grasped the 30-30 rifle with which he had killed himself. At their feet was the remains of a fire on which sat a kettle full of cut-up moose skin. Underneath the bodies was a sack containing spare duffle socks and Inspector Fitzgerald's diary. The following day the relief party came to a trail leading up a bank, and as they were feeling their way up it, they found a pair of snowshoes. At the top were the bodies of Fitzgerald and Carter. As Carter's face was covered with a handkerchief and his hands were placed upon his breast, it was evident that he had died first. Fitzgerald was lying near the fireplace.

Dempster carried on to Fort McPherson and reported the fatalities, and the next morning the police and some Gwich'in men retrieved the bodies and brought them to the village where they were given a military funeral. At an inquiry held to determine the cause of death, the commissioner said it was apparent that Inspector Fitzgerald had been hoping to make a fast journey and so cut down on rations to lighten the load, but as he had only recently returned from a patrol to Herschel Island, his dogs were tired and not up to peak performance. But most of the patrol's troubles resulted from not having a Gwich'in guide. Fitzgerald had instead relied on Carter who had only made the trip once previously, and that had been travelling in the reverse direction.

After reading the intriguing accounts of the Lost Patrol, I had been eager to see the trail to Dawson and in February 1970 was privileged to make the trip to Dawson City with Gwich'in men and see the confidence and ease with which they travelled in their country. Although there were times when I felt utterly cold and exhausted, and snowshoeing in minus fifty degrees took some of the romance away from our trip, not once did I lose confidence in my Gwich'in friends. We had deviated from the police patrol route because Andrew Kunnizzi, our chief guide, said that the Wind and the Little Wind River always had too much overflow and open water. From the Road River we had crossed the Eighty Mile Portage, passing the Rock River and the Eagle River, then over the head of the Peel River before roughly following the Blackstone River until we arrived at the fledgling Dempster Highway. Of all my travels in Gwich'in country, this patrol had demonstrated to me that the Gwich'in people had maintained their traditional heritage of survival in one of the harshest environments in North America.

When I stood in the Mission graveyard in 2009 and looked at the headstone and graves of the members of that patrol, it brought back memories of our patrol to Dawson City in 1970. But in re-enacting the journey of the Lost Patrol, our people were confident and sure of success. We didn't have a single compass between us, but unlike the police patrol, we had our Gwich'in guides and we went unerringly to our destination, 760 kilometres away in Dawson City. Afterwards, Stuart Hodgson, commissioner of the NWT from 1967 to 1979, wrote of our patrol that:

> *Few people in the world could carry off a dogsled journey on the scale of the Dawson Patrol so casually and yet with as much competence as the Loucheux (Gwich'in) people. One patrol member interviewed by a CBC reporter was asked why he was going. His reply: "I thought I'd like to see Dawson."*

After the 1930s and 1940s when travel had been frequent between the Hudson's Bay Company outposts such as Fort McPherson, Lapierre House, Destruction City, Dawson City, Old Crow and places on the coast, travel became centred around the Delta and the local mountains. However, after our centennial trip to Dawson City in 1970 and participation in a canoe pageant down the Fraser River, the old Gwich'in travel bug really seemed to take hold once again.

Although dog teams were falling out of fashion, with the advent of better communications, roads and snowmobiles, the Gwich'in started going farther afield once more because the people who were now elders in the settlement wanted to instill the knowledge of survival and travel into their young people. One adventurous group of half a dozen men made a trip to Faro by snowmobile, then an annual event was established to find and follow the old trail over the Richardson Mountains to Old Crow. Young people were encouraged to go on this trip and learn some bush survival skills en route.

CHAPTER SEVENTEEN

Across the Peel River and opposite the village ran the small creek that had been very familiar to Muriel and me because it led to Mary Firth's trapline, and in the mid-sixties I had built a small cabin about a kilometre from the river. Now, as Muriel and I walked north from the William Firth Health Centre, we wandered along the riverbank and saw a white canvas tent set on the opposite bank where "our" creek entered the Peel River, and in the eddy just north of the creek we could see floats that marked where a fishnet was set. Curious about who owned this tent, we inquired and learned that it belonged to Peter Firth, the youngest son of William and Mary. He had been a small, tousle-haired boy of about seven or eight years when we last saw him, but like everyone else he had grown, and when we met him we did not at first recognize him. But it was good to see that he was continuing the Gwich'in fishing tradition.

Many of the old ways had been changing even when Muriel and I were living in Fort McPherson. In the past, summer had been the time when the Gwich'in had been able to vary their diet of caribou meat with fresh fish and berries as they became available. At the fish camps they placed nets in the eddies and one or two men constructed fish wheels, ingenious contraptions that would scoop up fish and drop them into netted containers. They filleted the fish, slashed parallel lines into their sides and hung them up in the sun or

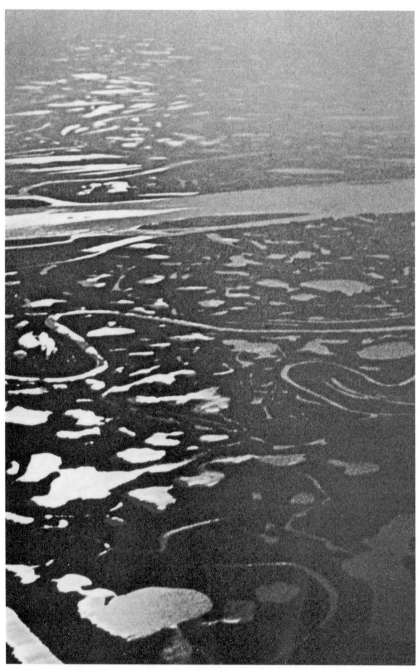

In the summer, the Gwich'in varied their diet with fish caught in the many lakes and rivers of the MacKenzie Delta.

a smokehouse to dry. Then they washed out the fish stomachs and poured fish roe or fish oil from burbot (locally called losh) into them before packing them into birchbark containers for winter use. Caribou hunting had been necessary to provide the community with meat, and in the old days the hunters would go out with their dog teams to places where they expected the huge caribou herds to be migrating. By the time we came to Fort McPherson, the people relied on the game warden to use a small plane to locate the herd, thus saving the hunters time and energy. Some of us who were not hunters would occasionally hire a plane that came to the settlement on some other business and then for an hour we would go looking for the caribou herds.

The use of dogs declined in the seventies, and as a result, the need for leather dog harness did too, but in the days when harnesses were needed for the hundreds of dogs in Fort McPherson and the cost of purchasing them from the store was prohibitive, they were made from anything that could be found that was strong enough. One woman, who must have had the strongest hand sewing machine in the country, sewed dog harness from some cast-off fire hose that she found at the garbage dump.

In the seventies the moose and caribou skin shelters that had been used for a hundred years or more were replaced with canvas tents made professionally in the local Canvas Tent Manufacturing facility, along with canvas packs and bags. Of course, the introduction of firearms had made a very welcome change from bows and arrows. But one old man, Christopher Colin, could still remember using bows and arrows out in the bush, and it was easy to see that he had been very proficient when he demonstrated the action of shooting one. When I asked him what the arrows had been like, he hand-carved a set for me, using raven feathers for the flights and tying them on with very thin sinew. He said he could not make the flint arrowheads anymore and so had put a small metal weight on one of the arrows to show me the crucial balance that was required.

I had been shown how to set a fishnet and for weeks in the summer I visited my net to get fish for my dogs and to give Muriel and me a break from canned food. Then William told us of a good place fairly close to the village where we could try setting a line for losh, a big ugly fish of the cod family that looked to me like a catfish. As they are bottom feeders, their large heads have barbels, which act as sensors to help the fish find its food. Their tapered bodies are known to reach over a metre in length, and some of the trappers caught them in order to use the large livers for mink bait in the winter.

William explained that the best time to catch them was overnight with a set line. Armed appropriately with large hooks, bait and some strong line, we walked down to Koe's Creek, and by the light of a large flashlight I baited the hooks and set them out at the mouth of the tiny creek. Not being a knowledgeable fisherman, I stood watching where the lines entered the water for a minute or two then we went home. Early the next morning I went down to the creek and pulled in the first line. Nothing. Pulled in the second line. Nothing again except that the bait was missing. Although not an enthusiastic fisherman, I am a great optimist and I experienced a feeling of hope (or was it desperation?) as I began hauling in the last line. This one felt different, heavier and sluggish, though there was none of the wild flinging and splashing one would expect from a hooked fish. Maybe a piece of driftwood? I pulled in the long line, and at last a greenish mottled head appeared and I landed a fair-sized losh, which seemed more dead than alive. I pushed a willow through its gills and carried it home to await William's advice, thinking that maybe he or Mary could use it for dog feed or mink bait.

It was several hours before I found time to take William to see my prize catch. It lay where I had left it on the ground, but then to my utter astonishment, as we stared at it, it started to move! It had been out of the water for two or three hours and it was still alive. William had seen the same thing happen even the day after one had been caught. He said he would be glad to take it, and having satisfied my losh-fishing desires, I was glad to see it go and never did set another hook for losh after that.

Fishing is something that is necessary when you are short of food, but I never had the patience to stand fishing for hours in the rain if I didn't have a bite within the first fifteen minutes. Then one summer I was up the Rat River and had taken a rod and line because I had heard that the water was clear and there was a good chance of catching some trout. My lures were minimal and after four of five casts I had managed to lose all but one. As I made one last cast, I saw the swirl of a large northern pike or jackfish close to some reeds on the riverbank, but it did not take the hook. Suddenly I was the one that was hooked and I wanted desperately to catch this big guy. I tried to pull in my line but to my disgust it had hooked on the bottom, and try as I might I could not get it free and finally lost my hook and lure altogether.

Okay, now my dander was up. I still had a hook or two though no lures, but looking around, I spied an empty oil can in the bottom of the canoe and used my sheath knife to cut a piece of tin from the lid. I then tied the shell casing from a .22 bullet to the piece of tin and last of all fastened a hook to this sad-looking affair. I cast to where I thought the pike might be, close to the reeds. Wham! He grabbed my homemade lure and after one or two struggles gave up—I think he felt sorry for me!—and let me pull him in like a piece of waterlogged wood. He didn't even struggle when I reached over and grabbed him by the gills and hoisted him into the canoe. If I had thought that this was what people got excited about, I would not have cast another line again, but later I had the experience of fishing for grayling when they were biting almost faster than I could throw my line in, and *that* was fishing!

Trying to make a better fisherman out of me, our teacher friend Mike Wiggins suggested that we take our dogs the several kilometres to Husky Lake above the Peel Plateau and try our hand at ice fishing. He had been told the lake had some good-sized fish in it and that we couldn't fail to catch some. We took a net, which we planned to set with the aid of a jigger, a wooden implement that could be made to crawl under the ice for the same length as the net. We would have to dig two holes to be able to set the net and then return in a day or two to check it. Thinking that it would make our work so much easier, I took along the long-bladed chainsaw that William used to cut ice blocks on the river. We went early in the morning to give us time to get to the lake, dig the holes, set the net and return by dark. The snow was deep, but the dogs did not have heavy loads and we arrived at Husky Lake after three hours of travel. We started by shoveling the snow from the surface and were soon standing on the ice. But the chainsaw wouldn't start. I pulled and pulled the starter rope until I was dripping with the effort. Then Mike tried but there was not even a peep from the saw.

"Okay, we'll do it the old way!" Mike picked up his axe and started a hole in the ice. I took over from him and by two in the afternoon we were down about a metre. Then taking it in turns we went down another sixty centimetres. There was still no sign of water, but we were getting a little nervous as we didn't know if there was only a few more centimetres of ice or another metre beneath where we were standing. But we did know that, as soon as we broke through, even if we didn't fall into the hole ourselves, it would quickly fill with water and we would be unable to set the jigger anyway. And even if we were able to get a net in, when we came back in a day or two, we would have to do all of this again because the hole would have frozen over. The final thing that convinced us to pack up and go home was the realization that this was only the first of the two holes that were necessary!

Obviously the Gwich'in knew something that we didn't know, which was why there were no Gwich'in fishnets at the lake. Perhaps we should have come a month or two earlier before the ice got too thick, and maybe we shouldn't have come at all!

CHAPTER EIGHTEEN

As Muriel and I drove east from Fort McPherson on the gravel Dempster Highway on our way to Tsiigehtch- ic, I found myself wondering which of the lakes to our left I had crossed back in the sixties when I travelled the sixty-two- kilometre dog team trail from Fort McPherson to Arctic Red River. Peter Firth, the youngest son of William and Mary Firth, told us that he still travelled the old route and that somewhere along it the dog team trail crossed the road, but it all looked so different now. Then as we neared Tsiigehtchic, I saw a large lake over to my right with several islands on it and I recognized it as Islands Lake, the last one before the old dog team portage that led to the village. On one of the points of land about three-quarters of the way down that lake was a lobstick, a tall tree with all of its branches cleared off to within the top couple of metres. From a distance such trees are quite notice- able, and this particular tree could be seen from the west end of the lake and acted as a guide toward the portage entrance. I had made that dog team journey many times, taking anywhere from eight to twelve hours. Now when the weather was good, the trip could be done by road in just over an hour, which was quite convenient but it left something missing.

The Dempster Highway wound down the hill toward the con- fluence of the Arctic Red River and the great Mackenzie River. To our right across the Arctic Red River we could see the buildings of

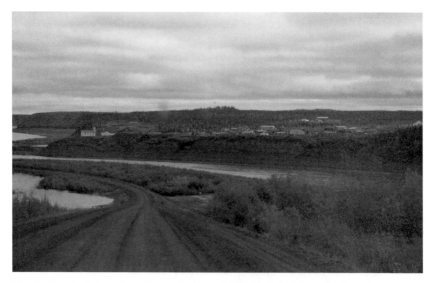

The Tsiigehtchic village is on the MacKenzie and Arctic Red rivers.

Tsiigehtchic, perched on a high bank overlooking both rivers. The houses were spread along the bank with the white painted Roman Catholic Church on a prominent point. The old Hudson's Bay Store stood at the top of the gravel road that climbed the hill from the dock, and behind it was the big new band store.

Straight ahead of us was the ferry, *Louis Cardinal*, that makes a three-way crossing from the Fort McPherson side of the Arctic Red to Tsiigehtchic and then over the Mackenzie River to meet the road leading north to Inuvik. The ferry was named after a very well-known and respected Metis RNWMP guide who had spent many afternoons in the later years of his life sitting on the porch of his house overlooking the Mackenzie River. Before he died at age ninety-five I had the good fortune to sit with him and listen to his stories of his days with the force. He had guided police patrols from Herschel Island to Dawson City and from Old Crow to Fort Good Hope, and I do believe that if he had not been on those patrols, many of them may have suffered the fate of Inspector Fitzgerald's 1911 patrol. In fact, Louis once told me that he had asked Fitzgerald to wait for him to return to Fort McPherson from another patrol

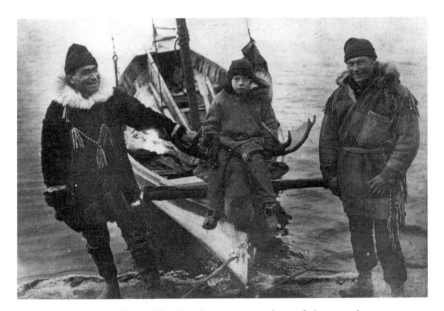

As a young man, Louis Cardinal was a member of the toughest summer patrol the RNWMP ever made. Here, he is with his son and an unnamed Mountie. ROSE CLARK PHOTO.

and then he would guide him to Dawson but Fitzgerald had been in a hurry and went without him.

It was Louis Cardinal who guided the second-ever Dawson to McPherson patrol in 1906, and he had been a member of the toughest summer patrol the RNWMP ever made, a trip that traced northern river routes all the way from Dawson City to Herschel Island on the Beaufort Sea. They had started from Dawson City in June, carrying their canoes when necessary. Sometimes they were up to their waists in water as they either lined the canoes up the fast-flowing rivers or held them back in the rapids. After negotiating the Peel River Canyon and then manoeuvring around a lot of submerged trees, they arrived safely in Fort McPherson and after a short rest paddled on to Aklavik and then Herschel Island.

On the return journey, as the patrol was about to leave Fort McPherson, the Hudson Bay factor, John Firth, advised them to stay as freeze-up was imminent, but the police wanted to get back. They decided to go back to Dawson via the Rat and Porcupine rivers, and if their luck held out they might catch the last paddlesteamer from Lapierre House, a Hudson's Bay Company outpost at the junction of the Bell and Water rivers.

They struggled against the current on the Rat River, spending days soaking wet and nights freezing cold, as the temperature dropped the higher they travelled into the mountains. Even when they finally arrived at Loon Lake, which is at the summit on the Yukon and NWT border, their difficulties were far from over. That night the temperature plummeted and when they woke the next morning they saw that ice covered the lake. They spent that day in camp but they were not prepared to winter at this elevation, and fortunately, the next day brought a chinook wind. They hastily packed up, and with one person breaking the mushy ice ahead of them with a pole, they paddled slowly until they came to the fast-running creek at the end of the lake. However, when they arrived at Lapierre House, they discovered the paddle steamer had left two days earlier, and they resigned themselves to spending the winter there. At least there was shelter and meat would be available from the Porcupine caribou herd that would be passing on their way north. Having accepted their lot, they were astounded the next morning to hear the whistle of the paddle steamer, which had returned to Lapierre House to make repairs after striking a deadhead, and with heartfelt thanks the patrol was able to board the boat. Fifty-two days after leaving Fort McPherson they arrived in Dawson City.

When he retired, Louis built a house for himself and Carolyn, his wife, just below the Hudson Bay property at Arctic Red River, and he situated it so he could sit on his porch in the sun, contentedly puffing on his pipe and reminiscing as he watched the Mackenzie River flow by. But he had another small cabin a few kilometres north of Arctic Red River on the east bank of the Mackenzie River where he and Carolyn spent leisurely weeks netting the rich waters and preparing dryfish for the winter.

I had passed his fishing camp several times when I had come to

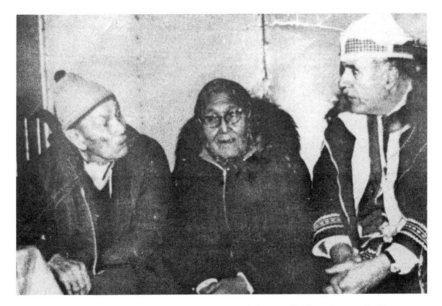

After he retired, Louis Cardinal, here with his wife Carolyn and Commissioner of the NWT Stuart Hodgson, lived on the Arctic Red River.

ROSE CLARK PHOTO.

Arctic Red River in my little aluminum boat, and what hair-raising trips they had been! Muriel and I had purchased the boat in the summer of 1967 after returning from a year at Dalhousie University. We thought it would be ideal for running up and down the Peel on short trips, especially now that we had two small children and we wanted to take them out without sacrificing them to the mosquitoes and black-flies. As a family we went down the Peel in our boat as far as the Mouth of the Peel but never ventured out onto the Mackenzie River itself. It was quite enjoyable making these quick trips, although I found that the water pump would quickly wear out in the abrasive muddy water. However, I became quite adept at changing the two metal plates on either end of the rubber impeller, an operation that involved breaking down the main shaft of the outboard motor, changing the worn parts, then putting it all back together again. In time I could accomplish this on the riverbank in twenty minutes, all the while swatting at mosquitoes, without losing any bolts or my temper.

Later that summer, I was due for my regular visit to Arctic Red River, and I decided it would be a good experience to travel there in my little speedboat. Loading the tiny craft had to be done carefully and the weight distributed evenly, otherwise the boat would plough through the water instead of rising onto the step as I increased the speed. I packed enough gas for a return journey, some extra oil and a tool kit, making sure that I had a spare propeller and several spare impeller plates.

It was calm at Fort McPherson when I set off, and going with the strong current, I soon left the settlement far behind. I passed the Husky Channel and started down the winding part of the Peel River before it reached its mouth. The water was quite high but the springtime debris had virtually vanished so the way was clear for me to have the motor going at full bore. But I began to worry as I approached the section of the river that had scared me when I had made a trip the previous spring in the long scow belonging to a Gwich'in man named Fred. We had come around a bend to see a huge whirlpool taking up the whole width of the river. The centre of the whirlpool looked to be two or three metres lower than the perimeter, and with some foreboding I saw quite a hole in the middle where logs and other flotsam were being sucked down. Fred, who was driving the scow from the rear, brought the scow over the lip of the whirlpool then, as we went around the top of the funnel, he waited until he was in line with the river again and gunned the motor, bringing us up and over the lip, much to my relief. Now as I came to this same place on the river, I was feeling rather tense and only relaxed when I saw that there was no longer a whirlpool. However, the fast water at this point was eroding the bank, and I kept away from it in case it collapsed.

At the Mouth of the Peel I stopped and visited for a short time with Jimmy Thompson, an elderly Gwich'in man, who advised me to be very careful on the Mackenzie River because a large sandbar had developed on the western side of the river where the Peel River came out. He instructed me to cross the Mackenzie right away and then follow the river up on the east shore until I got to Arctic Red River. I waved to Jimmy as I pulled away in my boat, but I felt very nervous because this was to be my first crossing of the Mackenzie River on my own, and as I saw the wide expanse of it before me, my boat seemed to shrink.

I moved out into the river, and as I turned toward the south, I could feel a slight wind behind me. Soon I could see the huge sand-bar, which seemed to stretch out almost halfway across the river, and I began edging my way around it. I did not want to get caught on the sand a long way from the shore because the wind from the north would make it difficult for me to push the boat off again. But as I motored further and further out into the Mackenzie, the waves be-gan to get higher and higher. Though the wind was not very strong, in that wide open space where the river was nearly two kilometres across, it was strong enough to curl the opposing current into huge breakers, and I was in the thick of it before I fully realized what was happening. My little boat was like a cork in the ocean, but I had to keep its nose facing into the current while at the same time edging out toward the other side of the river. My heart was in my mouth as I looked around me and saw that I was in one deep trough after another, and while I was in the bottom of these valleys, all I could see around me was water. By now I was wet with spray. I thought about heading for the sandbar, but the wind could have blown me into the shallow water where the kicker would have been no good, and I could have been stranded there. Going back to the Mouth of the Peel would have meant being broadside to the high waves as I turned, and I could easily have been swamped.

I sat tensely gripping the wheel with one hand and playing the throttle with the other, speeding up slightly as the boat climbed to the top of the trough and then decelerating as I slid down into the next one, feeling very cold but sweating at the same time. Sudden-ly I remembered that I had not put my life jacket on after leav-ing Jimmy Thompson's cabin, and I began feeling around for it and discovered I had been sitting on it! I edged it from under me and then, reluctantly letting go of the throttle for a moment, I carefully threaded one arm into the armhole while I held the wheel with the other. Then changing around to get the other arm in, I slowly managed to get it into place. However, fastening it would mean letting go of both the wheel and the throttle and I decided to leave well enough alone. In any case, I knew that if I was to be thrown into the water, I would not survive long enough to swim to shore, and the current would take me far down the river where it would be hard to reach any sort of shoreline.

Then almost imperceptibly the waves became smaller and I realized that I had crossed the worst of the deep water and was now in a relatively calm place. I glanced toward the shore and was surprised at how close it looked. While I was out in the middle of the river, I had only been aware of the huge waves around me. I nosed the boat toward shore and, landing on the beach, I stood uneasily on the slippery gravel. While still hanging onto the painter, I carried my Thermos to dry ground and had a cup of strong tea, which made me feel much better. Back in the boat, I started the outboard motor and turned up the Mackenzie River where I was once more aware how small my boat was as it sped up that wide expanse. I passed a tent frame on the bank, but seeing that the door was wide open and blowing in the breeze and there were no frames for drying fish or even any smoke, I knew no one was home. A little while later I saw smoke rising from a small log cabin, and as I drew closer, I saw a man sitting outside smoking a pipe. I immediately recognized the figure as that of Louis Cardinal. I turned the boat toward the shore and waved to him.

"Come up for tea!" he called, and I tied up the boat and climbed the bank to the cabin. Carolyn was behind the cabin slicing up a large cony, and she held up her fish-scale-soiled hands and apologized for being unable to shake my hand. Off to the side of the cabin there was a contraption that I recognized as a homemade wringer, which was being used to squeeze the moisture from a scraped and soaked moosehide that was being prepared for tanning. The moosehide was

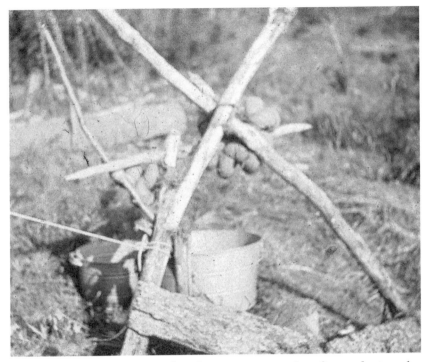

Moose skins were squeezed tight across a wooden frame during the tanning process.

all twisted up, and I could imagine the force that was required to get it that tight, and realized there was a lot of strength left in this old woman. Louis had already gone inside to put a kettle of water on the stove, and after putting a few pieces of firewood on top of the smoldering embers, he came back out and said, "Come and sit down. That water, it won't take long." Finding a chunk of cut log, I sat down by his side.

He wanted to know the condition of the river up by Point Separation and if I had seen any moose. I told him that there were no moose on the river when I came down, but I didn't admit to being scared stiff when I was crossing the Mackenzie. I don't think the words would have meant much to this great traveller. We talked for about an hour, enjoying strong cups of tea, then finally I told him that I must be on my way, although I would have gladly spent the rest of the day with the old man.

Past Louis' camp I saw two more tent frames beside the river, then up ahead I saw the village of Arctic Red River. I pulled into the dock at the foot of the village, tied the boat up and went up to the RCMP barracks where the corporal was expecting me. Joe Roenspiece was a very amiable policeman, though he was also someone you would want on your side in any disagreement. He came back down to the dock with me and, after we had secured my boat, helped carry my supplies up to his office. When we finally sat down, he gave me a list of all the people whose health he was worried about as well as the people who had asked to see me. When he explained that he would be busy that evening as he was expecting the arrival of a barge, I felt a wave of relief that it hadn't come earlier, because I would have had to contend with the waves *and* with the barge's wash.

I was with a patient when Joe knocked on the door to say the barge was in and he was going down to the dock. About an hour later, having seen my last patient, I wandered down to the river in the dark and met Joe coming up.

"I was just coming to get you," he said. "There's a guy on board who says he knows you. He's invited you down to their mess for coffee so I invited myself down there too."

"I don't know anyone who works on the boats," I said. "He must have me mixed up with someone else."

"He knew you were a nurse and that you lived in McPherson," Joe continued, "and it was only a coincidence that I mentioned your name when I was telling him about what was happening in the village."

"Well, let's go and find out. I haven't met anyone on a boat since I was in the merchant navy," I said, "and that's a *long* time ago!"

These tugs, which pushed their "tows" ahead of them, would nose them up against the dock or the shore, depending where they wanted to land their cargoes. The tow itself was like a large floating dock, loaded down with freight for different communities along the river. So now we went down to the dock, jumped onto the tow and walked along its considerable length, past huge piles of freight, until we could see the lights in the topmost cabin of the *Pelican Rapids*, which was tied up directly behind its tow. I reached the end of the tow first and was preparing to jump down onto the deck of the *Pelican* when a swirl of white water stopped me in my tracks. I had just assumed that the bow of the *Pelican* was as wide as the tow's stern and had almost jumped down into the river.

"Careful!" Joe called, grabbing my coat. "Don't fall in there! It's over eighteen metres deep with a very strong current. We'd never find you!"

With the feeling that the Mackenzie River was being a bit hostile to me, I climbed carefully down onto the boat. As we made our way to the mess cabin, I silently thanked my guardian angel for that swirl of white water.

In the cabin a rather small young man got up and greeted me, and I felt very apologetic because he did not look at all familiar to me. "My grandmother, Winnie Hiley, who lives in Calgary, knows you," he said, "and when she found out that I was coming up here on the *Pelican*, she told me to be sure to look you up. She even showed me a picture so I would recognize you!"

Ah, it all made sense now. My wife and I had met Winnie at a church conference in Vernon some time back and she had kept tabs on us through a mutual friend. Now, after catching me up on his grandparent's health, he showed us around the boat and I was impressed by its compactness and cleanliness. We had several cups of coffee and a good talk, and as we left, Joe remarked, "It just goes to show, doesn't it, what a small world we live in, especially up here in the Territories!" This reminded me of a letter I had received from Britain addressed to "Keith Billington, NWT, Alaska." As mortified as I was at the ignorance of the sender who thought that the Northwest Territories were in Alaska, I was more amazed that the post office was so tuned in that they could find me in this vast expanse of tundra!

Several days later after doing physicals on all the youngsters in Arctic Red River's one-room school, then tuberculin testing the children and some of their parents, visiting the elders and seeing the one expectant mom in the village—or at least the only one admitting it at the time—I got ready to leave in my little boat. I packed every-thing, put on my life jacket and tied it securely. I was filled with a mixture of elation, excitement and downright fear as I set off down the east side of the river.

Once more the weather was calm, the sun was out, and I kept fairly close to the shore where there was no sign of waves. Louis Cardinal's camp was quiet as he and Carolyn had come to Arctic Red for some supplies, but as I neared the Mouth of the Peel River I could feel myself tensing up. It's one thing to go head-on into large waves, but I absolutely detested going through waves when they were going in my direction because they pushed my little boat's stern to one side so the outboard motor would not react properly to the helm. At times like this the boat could easily be washed side-ways, the next wave would swamp it and that would be it for me.

Slowly I moved out toward the middle of the river where the current was strong and the water swirled and swished like a seeth-ing caldron. This fearful situation was made worse by the waves that lifted the small boat high one moment, with me hanging on to the wheel tightly, and then plunged it down into the depths the next. Meanwhile, the waves coming from behind seemed determined to make the boat corkscrew around, and I had difficulty in keeping it headed north while at the same time edging it over to the west side of the river. And then came the few fearful moments when the strong current from the Peel River wanted to push me back out into the Mackenzie again, and I thought about the impeller and hoped that it would not let me down at this critical moment.

But I made it through and pulled into bank below Jimmy Thompson's cabin. The whole place was deserted now, but I went into the empty cabin and had some lunch. When at last I felt my nerves were under control again, I hoisted the rear of the boat onto the shore, changed the impeller plates as a preventive measure and headed for home without incident.

After this adventure, with its alternating fear and adrenaline rushes, had passed into the back recesses of my memory, I made several more trips to Arctic Red River in my little speedboat, and each time when I approached the Mackenzie River, I would chastise myself for going, but the excitement and dread was like a drug that I couldn't shake off.

❄   ❄   ❄

Before our children were born, Muriel and I had taken turns going to Arctic Red River either by dog team or the Otter. The first time Muriel went was by dogsled and we had no idea how long it would take or what it was like to travel by that mode. John Simon had been hired to drive the dogs and Muriel would ride in the carriole. She was all bundled up and waiting for John to arrive when William Firth came in and said in surprise, "Don't you know it's forty below? It's going to be really cold for you."

"I'll be okay, William. I've got my big sleeping bag to lie in and a couple of hot water bottles."

William was not convinced but didn't say anything else, and when John arrived with his dog team, William carried Muriel's supplies out and I tucked them into her sleeping bag. She then climbed into the toboggan and I placed the hot water bottles around her and she certainly looked cozy enough.

"Ask the RCMP to call the detachment here when you arrive," I told her. She waved, John spoke to his dogs and they went out of the yard in a flurry of flying snow. That evening the police came by to say that Muriel and John had arrived safely. It had taken them about nine hours, and Muriel was staying with the DeWitts, the schoolteacher and his wife.

I didn't hear anything more until two days later when Muriel walked into the nursing station with a very pink face from the cold and stood by the stove to warm herself.

"How was it?" I asked, putting the kettle on for a hot drink.

"It was fun on the way there, but very cold coming back as we were driving into the wind. John made us some tea at the police cabin because I'd finished the Thermos."

William came to visit as soon as he heard that Muriel was back and had a coffee with us while Muriel ate a late supper and gave us a detailed account of her trip. William seemed very relieved. He wanted us both to enjoy the northern way of life, but because we were so inexperienced, he was always worried in case we came to harm.

Most of the subsequent trips that Muriel made to Arctic Red River were by plane, which she said was much more comfortable and quicker. As the scheduled plane came to Fort McPherson on Monday, Wednesday and Friday but only went weekly to Arctic Red, she would go on the scheduled flight to Arctic Red and then side-charter it off its scheduled run so she could get back. But I preferred the more adventurous way. The first few times I went to Arctic Red River by dog team, William Teya took me with his dogs, which was okay in many ways, but like a teenage driver I wanted to do it by myself. So, with a lot of encouragement from William Firth, and the use of his dog team, at last I went on my own, confident that I could find the way.

I did well until I came to a new seismic road that I didn't know existed. As a result, I travelled for hours in what I thought was the wrong direction, then turned around and followed the traditional but unused dog team trail. One of the dogs I had borrowed from William died. I then got lost and had to spend the night sleeping in my carriole, but when it got light I realized where I had gone wrong and finally arrived in Arctic Red River just as the corporal from the detachment was setting out to search for my frozen corpse.

After that almost disastrous trip I travelled that route many times over the years without having a problem, but my visits were not without incident. On one trip I took Old Chief Johnny Kay's team and it was a pleasure to run his dogs, which were all very well behaved and worked well, exactly what I would expect of a team from this exceptional man. The journey was not fast but it was steady, and I arrived there feeling tired as usual after jogging on and off for several hours behind the dogs. As I was invited to stay with the corporal and his wife, I drove the team into their yard and was greeted by a cacophony of barks and howls from the numerous dogs in their large fenced-off corral. These dogs were all part of the RCMP sled dog breeding program and were sent all over the Arctic from there. My dogs were not impressed, and even though they held their tails high, their senses were on full alert and they glanced around them uneasily.

Joe Masazumi, a very friendly Japanese/Slavey Native special constable who was married to a quiet Slavey woman from Fort Good Hope, met me in the yard and waved me over to an area where my dogs could be tied. "Just tie them here and I will feed them for you," he said and he walked off to get some feed, his slight frame moving easily among his dogs. (Joe and his wife made an odd-looking couple as he was small boned and his Japanese genes showed very prominently whereas she was a lot taller and heavier.)

I tied up my dogs and went to the corporal's house and was soon was being entertained by his two small children, who were very lively and full of mischief. "You know, Keith," Margaret, the corporal's wife, told me, laughing as she indicated her four-year-old, "this little monkey put one of the pups into the dryer yesterday, but luckily he was too small to reach the controls!"

A few minutes later there was a knock on the door, and Margaret came to say, "It's Joe. Your dogs have got loose."

Joe was apologetic as he told me that, after one of my dogs got loose, several of the others had pulled their stakes up as well, and he was worried they might get into his dog pens and cause a riot. The RCMP dogs were all Siberians, and though they could be as noisy as any other dog, they were not as aggressive as the Mackenzie River huskies I was driving, but they would defend themselves in a fight. Joe was reluctant to handle the dogs I had brought until he knew their dispositions, but when I explained that they were Johnny Kay's dogs, he said, "Oh, Johnny's dogs! I'll catch them okay then. You go back to the house." And with that, he cornered one and then another and fastened them to some trees away from the RCMP dogs.

Joe was an expert dog handler and had travelled long distances with his dogs, and he and the corporal took teams out at regular intervals during the week to keep the dogs in good condition. On one occasion Joe had been busy in the dog yard when to his amazement a large wolf paused on the perimeter of the yard. Wolves are very shy of humans and human habitations, but this one stayed to sniff around, and Joe thought that maybe he was an old one and had been drawn by the smell of the dog feed, especially to the pit fish, which always gave off quite an aroma. Slowly Joe moved toward the office where the rifles were kept, grabbed a rifle and some ammunition and headed out again. Rabies was endemic in the North at that time and he was not taking any chances. By now the wolf had moved closer to the dog pens and the police dogs were running around sniffing the air. They didn't like what they could sense but could not see. Aiming carefully, Joe fired and was relieved to see the wolf drop. Using some heavy gloves, he dragged the wolf over to a place where he could burn it, glad that Margaret's children had been playing safely in the house when the wolf had visited.

On another one of my visits I was in the kitchen drinking coffee—a favorite occupation of nurses and police—when right below us on the lawn a big black bear sauntered past, stopping to sniff the side of the house and in no hurry at all. The corporal went to get his rifle and, telling me to stay indoors, he went carefully outside. A few minutes later there was a loud report as he fired once, then again. "It's not going to be wandering around here anymore," he told me when he returned and pointed to where it lay at the edge of the property. "He walked right by the place where my children are usually playing and that wouldn't be funny!" His wife and children had fortunately left for Inuvik on the plane that morning.

Joe Masazumi looked after my dogs every time I stayed in Arctic Red River, for which I was very thankful, and when I was ready to leave, he had them all hitched up by the time I came out of the house. After one such visit, he told me just before I started off, "Dale Clark said that if you call by his place on your way, he has a load of stick fish for you." Dale was a hard worker, the son-in-law of Louis Cardinal and, though not a blood relative, he had the same work ethic. He sometimes took on jobs for the Bay, served as the school janitor, hunted and trapped and then still found time to set nets for the fish that his wife prepared.

Stick fish—also called crooked backs—are small (only about one and a half kilograms) but because they are very bony, they were used in those days almost exclusively for dog feed. They were skewered through their gills with a stick, ten at a time, and hung up to freeze or thrown into a pit dug into the frozen ground in the fall.

Dale and Rose, his wife, lived on a hillside close to the road that I was to leave by, but I had difficulty halting the dogs at their house because they were well fed, rested and eager to run on the trail and I had an almost empty toboggan. I had to tie the headliner to a post while Dale filled up my toboggan with ten racks of fish, enough to feed my dogs for a couple of weeks. "That'll slow them down a bit for you," Dale said with a laugh, and how right he was! I asked him how much he wanted for the fish, and to my surprise he answered, "Nothing. It's because you come to visit us with your dogs. Not many white people travel the country like we do anymore."

I wasn't sure if he was just being polite and generous because I was still fairly new to the North, so I thanked him profusely and shook his hand in the Gwich'in way, with one firm shake of the hand. Pulling their heavy load, the dogs careened down the rest of the hill, crossed the river and went up the hill opposite Arctic Red River. I knew it was going to be a slow journey but I was thankful that I had such a good team that was equal to the challenge.

❄   ❄   ❄

It seems that tempting fate was something I had to do periodically. Early one winter I ran the risk of getting lost—as I had on my very first solo dog team trip—when I decided to try to be the first to travel by dog team to Arctic Red River. I would skirt all the lakes because the ice was not yet thick enough to cross them, and instead follow the seismic roads with neither map nor compass to guide me. A friend, Ted Haas, was interested in a little adventure so I asked him to accompany me. As this was to be the first trip of the year for the dogs, we did not expect too much from them—and the same went for us, too. We expected it would take about two days to make the journey and packed food and supplies accordingly.

We travelled north along the first seismic road we came to, following our instincts. The temperature was a bit warm for the dogs, hovering around minus six degrees (C), and the sky was overcast, but our toboggans glided quite well over the several centimetres of snow. I could remember seeing a seismic road heading east marked on someone's map, so after travelling for a few hours we took the first one we saw, turning right and heading east with all the naive confidence in the world. We left a well-defined trail behind us and I knew that it would be visible for a long time unless we had a heavy snowfall.

We went on, zigzagging from one road to another as they skirted close to various lakes, but generally we kept to what I felt was an easterly direction, and I was confident that we were well on our way. Then suddenly the road that we were following came to an abrupt end at the edge of a long narrow lake and we were faced with the prospect of forcing our way through thick bush all around the lake or crossing the ice. Neither choice excited me, so I did what any Englishman would do in the circumstances—I made a fire and a pot of tea.

Later while Ted made supper, I took out my binoculars and looked around. There was something on the other side of the lake that looked unnatural, and the more I looked the more I was convinced that it was a fresh dog team trail or perhaps a snowmobile trail. If it was, it meant that we were close to some habitation, and as we had been travelling for about seven hours, it could possibly be a camp. Unfortunately, the overcast sky hid the sun completely while we had been switching from one cut line to another, and we hadn't been able to use it to guide us. Since it was now getting dark, we tied up the dogs for the night. The night being warm, we decided that an open camp would suffice, so we made ourselves some spruce bough beds and rolled out our thick sleeping bags. I told Ted that in the morning after an early breakfast I wanted to test the ice to see if we could cross this narrow lake and not have to go back over our old trail.

I awoke twice in the night, once after a vivid dream, which I could not remember the next morning, and a second time after the dogs began howling in unison. Could they hear wolves with their keen hearing? I lifted a corner of the sleeping bag and listened intently once the dogs had quietened, but I couldn't hear anything. My face was cold and it felt a bit wet so I wiped my beard with the back of my hand, pulled my toque over my ears and went back to sleep. After what seemed only like a few more minutes I squinted as daylight intruded through a crack in my sleeping bag. I threw back the covers and was amazed to see that it was snowing heavily. My sleeping bag had about ten centimetres of snow on it, and when I glanced over at Ted, I could see his slowly moving form under his own blanket of snow. I pulled the sleeping bag slowly back over me and snuggled down while I chewed on this new development.

A little while later I heard Ted's exclamation of surprise as he woke and saw our winter wonderland. "Hey Ted," I called from underneath my covers. "Are you going to make breakfast this morning?"

He laughed. "I was just sitting up to see if you had made it yet!"

I suggested that we break camp and eat later. The way it was snowing made me concerned that if we had to follow our trail back we might not see it under all of this new snow, and we might find ourselves well and truly lost in the Delta. The seismic crews had been all over the place leaving their lines so the whole terrain looked like a chequered flag. We soon had everything packed and the dogs hitched up to the loaded sleds and I led the way down to the icy lake. I took one careful step, then another. The ice held!

I signaled to the dogs to come down and they came, though they looked pensively at the ice. I held my leader's collar when he reached me and then took another step. Crack! Without warning my foot went through the ice, soaking my leg but with some relief my mukluk touched bottom. I shouted to Ted, who was watching with a worried look on his face, that all was okay, my voice projecting a confidence that I did not feel. I walked out steadily toward the centre of the narrow lake with the dogs following literally at my heels. I would have preferred them to stay behind a bit and spread the weight around but I don't think they wanted to be left all alone out on the ice. They also seemed to sense that this was not a good time to get all tangled up and start a fight, and as they walked on steadily their ears were perked up as though they were listening for the ice to crack.

With considerable relief I reached the shore and yelled through the heavily falling snow for Ted to follow. His dogs whooshed down on to the lake eager to catch up, and I had only started to change my wet mukluk when they arrived. But as I finished changing, I looked around at the trail that was fast disappearing under the new snow, and then suddenly I wasn't worried about losing the trail anymore. I knew where we were.

"Guess what, Ted?"

"What?"

"See this dog team trail just here?" I pointed at the only trail around. "This leads directly to Fort McPherson!"

"How do you know that?"

"Because we made it yesterday morning! Can you remember when we were following the seismic road for a short way then we turned around because it didn't feel right? Somehow we have made one giant circle and fortunately we didn't get lost."

Ted looked up at the dark clouds and the heavy snow. "I think maybe we should head back home while we still can." I agreed.

As they always did, the dogs seemed to sense that we were heading home, and they just flew along the trail. As we pulled into the village, the snow stopped, but we were glad to be home and on firm footing. My next trip to Arctic Red River would have to wait until the traditional trail was safe to go on.

❆ ❆ ❆

I would normally travel to Arctic Red by dog team in eight to twelve hours, depending upon trail and snow conditions, but when Corporal Shane Hennan called to say he was thinking of making a patrol to Arctic Red River on one of the RCMP's two new Snowcruisers and asked if I would like to join him, I said, "Yes!" and then qualified this by adding, "if I can borrow a snowmobile," as there were not many in the village at that time. Until then I had been stubbornly resisting the Mounties' argument that snowmobiles were cheaper and quicker than dogs, preferring the advice of the old men who said knowingly, "Ah, you can't eat a Skidoo, and if it breaks down you can't carry it in the sled like you can when a dog gets sick!" On the other hand, I had to concede that you did not have to feed a snowmobile during the summer.

However, as I was due to travel to Arctic Red River on my monthly visit, the corporal's invitation was very timely. I spoke with Walter Alexie, who was a mechanic at the Northern Canada Power Commission and one of the few long-time employees and wage earners in the village. He owned a Bombardier Elan snowmobile and was willing to rent his machine to me for two or three days because he would be at work most of that time. He told me the correct mix of gas and oil to use and I topped up the snowmobile's tank and packed an extra can in my dog toboggan that would pull easily behind the snowmobile. I also packed the few supplies needed to stock the medical cupboard that we maintained in the RCMP barracks at Arctic Red River. I added my usual medical kit, which was well wrapped up in my Three Star sleeping bag, plus some food in case we stopped on the way, and I was ready to go on this first quick trip by snowmobile.

We left at seven in the morning and within an hour we were speeding over a long portage and making record time. I was ahead and going full out when I dropped off the portage onto a lake and had gone no more than twenty metres when I felt the drag of overflow, stopped the snowmobile and stepped into about thirty centimetres of water. Shane saw the danger as he came to the edge of the lake, stopped his machine in time and came to help me. Two hours later we had pulled the snowmobile to the shore, both of us sweating heavily and both with soaking wet feet. We turned the snowmobile over and hacked at the now frozen slush on the track and the wheels. Then we surveyed our position. If we tried to carry on along the dog team trail, we knew there would be another few dozen lakes to cross, and if they had overflow on them, they would be impossible to cross. Shane knew of a seismic or survey road that went a few kilometres out of the way but skirted all of the lakes, so we retraced our trail until we found the seismic road and turned onto it. Twenty kilometres out we came across our first obstacle, a running creek that had cut a swath right across the road—and this in the middle of winter, too! We cut trees and made a very narrow bridge and then Shane mounted his snowmobile, and gunning it, crossed the makeshift bridge safely. I followed him in seconds, relieved to be on the other side without tipping over.

We reached a point where we had to turn off onto a trail that had been cut as a winter works project, but unfortunately for us it was cut in late winter when the snow was deep and now the stumps protruded about forty-five centimetres above the present snow level. We managed to manoeuvre around most of these, and where this was impossible we lifted, pushed and pulled the machines over them.

Just when I thought nothing else could go wrong, the Elan engine coughed, choked and died. Any love I might have been developing for a snowmobile died with the engine. Even a swift kick only hurt the kicker, and the machine just sat there without a response. Shane, a mechanical genius, took the carburetor apart, quickly cleaned it, reassembled it and we were off again, only to have the same problem occur minutes later. Shane fixed the same part four times in the next hour, and I was glad to see that he finally got so frustrated that he kicked the snowmobile before saying that the gas can must have more dirt in it than gas.

When we came to Frog Creek, called Neyendo Creek by the Gwich'in, a narrow winding stream at the bottom of a steep gully, we slithered to a stop at the bottom of the hill. I threw a frozen lump of shale onto the ice to test it and watched with disappointment as it broke through and disappeared, leaving a widening black hole. Shane then drove along the creekside, found a place that looked narrow enough and shot over to the other side as fast as he could. I followed and went through some soft ice on the far side of the creek but it wasn't enough to cause me any problems. We then had to help each other drive and push the snowmobiles up the bank to the top of the gully, by which time we were sweating and exhausted so we stopped for some tea and supper.

As we ate our sandwiches in the quietness, we discussed the pros and cons of snowmobiles, and not surprisingly the cons still outweighed the pros at this moment! However, I started to feel cold as the knees of my wind pants were wet from kneeling on the snowmobile seat and now were becoming hard-crusted with ice, so we shattered the peace as the engines roared into life again. We had travelled on uneventfully for several kilometres when I heard a loud bang behind me and a shout from Shane, whose snowmobile ski had struck a hidden tree stump. The ski was broken and the only way we could continue was by tying the two skis on his machine together at the front and back and hoping that there were no other obstacles hiding just underneath the snowy surface to catch the rope that was tying the skis. This situation became more hazardous because we were soon driving in the dark, the snowmobile lights jumping up and down as we crossed the bumpy terrain.

Just when we were thinking that this trail must go on forever, we were delighted to see three snowmobile lights heading toward us, and soon we were telling our tale of woe to the corporal from Arctic Red River, the Bay manager and Dale Clark, who had come to look for us. Now we chugged along in a convoy to arrive in the village a short time later. Our exhaustion evaporated as we talked and laughed about this "quick trip" that we had completed. It was late when we finally crawled into our sleeping bags in the RCMP barracks.

Early the next morning I filled up the medical cupboard and then went to see several older people who had left messages for me. When I returned to the barracks, I loaded up ready for the return journey. I looked forward to the trip with a mixture of excitement and dread, especially after Shane, having conferred with Dale Clark, said that we would try a different route back so we would not have to travel over the stumpy trail. It was a circuitous seismic trail of an estimated ninety-six kilometres that would bring us out slightly northwest of Fort McPherson and from there we should be able to pick up a dog team trail. There was only one creek marked on the map, the only place that might give us problems.

We soon found the seismic trail where the snow was quite deep and untrammeled, with not even an animal track to be seen. Shane led the way, his repaired skis slicing through the virgin snow. We kept the snowmobiles going at full speed and the trail ahead of us rolled on endlessly. But all good things come to an end, and my heart sank as my engine died and the sound of Shane's machine drifted off into the distance. Then a moment of inspiration came to me and I checked the gas tank. Empty! I was almost glad except that Shane was carrying all the spare gas in his toboggan. I sat and waited and after ten minutes I heard the sound of his returning snowmobile. Twenty minutes later we were off again and we didn't stop until we arrived at the creek. It wasn't as small as we had hoped and with dismay we saw that there was a thirty-metre stretch of ice to cross. Going as fast as we could, we both roared over the ice and only when we reached the other side did we look back. Then we saw two very wet trails snaking across the ice where water was already seeping over them.

It was dark by the time we saw the first dogsled trail and knew that we were close to home. As we got closer to the village we saw the welcoming street lights. The ride back had been quite exhilarating, but when I thought about it and talked to Muriel about the trip, I realized that I had missed the companionship of the dogs and the feeling of security I had when I was travelling with them. It was one of those first-hand experiences that illustrated the conflict between the old and the new way of life.

EPILOGUE

REMINISCING IS USUALLY AN OLD PERSON'S game. After all, if you are going to think back you must have had some experiences to think back on. Our return trip to Fort McPherson in 2009 certainly gave Muriel and me an opportunity to think back, but it also gave us the opportunity to compare the modern village and its residents with the village and the people that we had known back in the sixties. We looked at these things not with a view to deciding which one was better. Although people talk about "the good old days," in reality they were often not so good, and the people who think they were have let the good memories obliterate the bad ones. Sure, there were the good days when the sun shone down out of a cloudless sky, the caribou were close and plentiful and the fishnets were full. But then there were the days of hauling wood and water, battling the freezing temperatures in a tent, watching babies and other family members die because of the isolation and lack of services, and freezing fingers during days and nights on the trapline trying to make a living.

It is a romantic past but not a terribly desirable one.

As we drove up the Dempster Highway, we saw heavily laden trucks bringing supplies. We wandered around the stores and saw fresh produce. California grapes 160 kilometres inside the Arctic Circle! What luxury! What a price! People were riding around in pick-up trucks and on quad bikes, and we heard the turbo-prop planes landing at the year-round airport twice a day. Changes and improvements. But it was the people who made all of these things happen. The Gwich'in people have adjusted to their new way of living and still have retained many of their old ways, the ways that count, the way that they treat each other and the people from Outside. There is no longer a Fleming Hall Hostel in Fort McPherson, and the schoolchildren do not have to go to Inuvik for higher education. They can finish their grade 12 right at the modern, large Chief Julius School.

Does everyone now get on with their fellow Gwich'in brothers and sisters? No, they are human beings and subject to the same weaknesses as all of us—jealousy, anger, pride and the host of other human emotions—but these negative things are kept in check by the leadership of strong people like Mary Teya and the members of a strong band council, most of whom were still youngsters when we first knew them. It is humour, generosity, friendliness and the ability to accept people for what they are that most Gwich'in people have demonstrated every day of their lives, and this is what Muriel and I were delighted to find during our return visit to Fort McPherson.

We stayed for a week, certainly not long enough to be authorities on the changes there, but we couldn't help but notice the general overall improvements. We visited families unannounced and were welcomed with the old courtesy and something that was almost unheard of forty years ago—a hug! People are now able to demonstrate their emotions. We were stopped on the road and asked to go into houses to visit, and many messages were brought to us asking for us to stop by to see some of the older people.

In the week that we wandered around Fort McPherson we saw only one intoxicated person on the road and that was from a distance. We heard that alcohol and drugs are a problem in the settlement, but is there somewhere in North America where they are not a problem? The Gwich'in Tribal Council, under the able leadership of Freddy Carmichael, who had regained his Gwich'in heritage, has spent millions of dollars on rehabilitation. They have built a beautiful self-contained building close to Inuvik, but without any direct access to the town, where the Gwich'in people can go to recover from the physical and mental effects of substance abuse and then relearn their old ways. The unique aspect of this program is that when people are discharged from this unit, they are sent to stay at a traditional camp in the bush where they are taught by elders about their culture in a very practical and meaningful way.

We were saddened by the number of deaths that had occurred; disease amongst the middle-aged and older people and violence and accidents amongst the young have all taken their toll. But interestingly enough, the major cause of death in all age groups was cancer, and we can only wonder what is causing this high incidence. In spite of the large number of young and vibrant people in the community today, the population has not increased substantially in the last forty years. In 1965 there was a total population of 852 in the village; by 1995 it had dropped to approximately 800 people and it is still about the same even today.

Water and sanitation systems have improved tremendously, as have housing and roads. Our old nursing station is long gone, replaced twice in the past thirty years as the needs of the people became apparent and as the responsibility for health moved from the federal government to the government of the Northwest Territories in Yellowknife. Staffing in the Health Centre has increased over 200 percent of what it was, and the nurse-in-charge is no longer an Outsider, having been there for over nine years, working side by side with two Gwich'in registered nurses and another nurse plus other visiting professional staff.

The North has become a mecca for people who enjoy living history, vast expanses of untouched wilderness and a sense of adventure. As we travelled the Dempster Highway, we stopped at Rock River and Eagle Plains, places that have a valuable Gwich'in history, places that we had visited by dogsled as a family and where I had travelled with Gwich'in men as they hunted caribou or took part in the last real McPherson to Dawson dog team trip in 1970. They looked different from the modern perspective of a powerful truck and trailer, seeing them from the gravel road, but though it was much easier travelling, it somehow felt wrong to be speeding down the highway instead of travelling at the slow and steady pace of a dog team. However, we were delighted to find that the Dempster Highway was not overcrowded, that there was virtually no dust and that there were very few large transport trucks on the road.

We have all changed and will continue to change, but the North remains a vast, wonderful, beautiful, magnificent and exciting land, and if I was Gwich'in, I would be very satisfied and proud that it was my home.

ENDNOTES

1. Slobodin, Richard. "How the People Learned About Money." Offprint from *Polar Notes*, Stefansson Collection June 1963.

2. Clairemont, Donald. "Deviance Amongst Indians and Eskimo in Aklavik, N.W.T." Donald Clairemont NCRC-63-9 October 1963, page 9.

3. Willis, J.S. (MD, DPH, General Superintendant, Northern Health Services, Indian and Northern Health.) "Mental Health in the North." 1959. Introduction, chapter 1, and page 4, chapter 2.

4. Boag, Dr. T.J. "The White Man in the Arctic. A Preliminary Study of Problems of Adjustment." *The American Journal of Psychiatry*, December 1952, page 109:6.

5. Slobodin, Richard. "Band Organization of the Peel River Kuchin." National Museum of Canada Bulletin No. 179. Anthropological Series No. 55.

ACKNOWLEDGEMENTS

This book could not have seen the light of day without the able assistance of the publisher and staff at Harbour Publishing. Anna Comfort has been very encouraging along the way, as has Rachel Page. I would especially like to thank Betty Keller who as a skillful editor was able to see what I was trying to say and made me say it.

The Gwich'in people of Fort McPherson and Tsiigehtchic have shown how they have successfully adapted to new ways and Mary Teya, a community elder, remains a dear friend.

My thanks to Frank Dunn, RCMP (retired), for the use of some of his photographs.

Lastly, I want to thank my wife, Muriel, who patiently shared the exciting and stimulating Arctic life and who continues to encourage me daily.